# THE UNITED STATES NAVY SEALS WORKOUT GUIDE

# THE UNITED STATES
# NAVY SEALS
# WORKOUT GUIDE

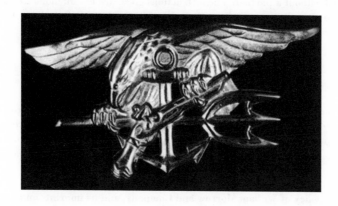

## THE EXERCISE AND FITNESS PROGRAMS BASED ON THE U.S. NAVY SEALS AND BUD/S TRAINING

## COMMAND MASTER CHIEF DENNIS C. CHALKER, U.S.N. (RET.),
### WITH KEVIN DOCKERY

WILLIAM MORROW AND COMPANY, INC.

NEW YORK

This publication is not officially endorsed by the U.S. Navy or any of its Commands.

This program is designed for people who are in good health. There may be risks involved in connection with some of the exercises in this book so they should not be completed without a partner. The instructions given are not intended as a substitute for qualified medical counseling. Consult your physician before doing this or any other exercise routine.

Library of Congress Cataloging-in-Publication Data

Chalker, Dennis C.
The United States Navy SEALs workout guide : the exercise and
fitness programs based on the U.S. Navy SEALs and BUD/S training /
Command Master Chief Dennis C. Chalker with Kevin Dockery.—1st  ed.
p.   cm.
ISBN 0-688-15862-5
1. Exercise.   2. Physical fitness.   3. United States. Navy.
SEALs.   I. Dockery, Kevin.   II. Title.
GV481.C517   1998
613.7'1—dc21          97-35393
CIP
Printed in the United States of America

First Edition

1   2   3   4   5   6   7   8   9   10

BOOK DESIGN BY OKSANA KUSHNIR

www.williammorrow.com

To the men of the Teams:
Those who went before and whose sacrifices paved the way,
the Teammates who led, followed, and fought
alongside me during my career,
and to those future generations of SEALs yet to come.
For them this book is dedicated.

# AUTHOR'S NOTE

U.S. Navy Special Warfare represents a professional unit of men with backgrounds in all walks of life. The public knows us as the Navy SEALs, but to ourselves, we are all members of the Teams. To be a part of the Teams takes self-motivation, pride in yourself, an attitude of not even considering giving up, the ability to function as a member of a team, and patience. BUD/S (Basic Underwater Demolition/SEAL) is where you will take these traits and forge them into an unbreakable will. These abilities will stay with you for the balance of your Navy career as well as the rest of your life.

BUD/S teaches an individual to think positively, work as a Teammate, and always strive to win. You will also learn that the only easy day was yesterday, and that is only because it's already over. Quality is what makes the SEALs what they have been, are today, and will remain for the future. And all members of the Teams began developing their quality in training.

Once you have passed training and are in the Teams, you will have to prove yourself a warrior. Many challenges will be tasked to you, challenges that you will strive to meet or exceed. The terms "I can't" or "I will not" are not part of a SEAL's vocabulary; they are not even thought of. Every member of the Teams is a brother, and in this brotherhood, we take care of our own and always help each other when problems arise. Although this brotherhood can be found in many organizations, particularly those where men face danger together, nowhere is it stronger then in the Teams.

The longer an individual remains in the Teams, the better he will succeed at life when he finally leaves. I've seen many SEALs retire and make their second lives even more successful than when they were in the Navy. It is the positive attitude of always striving to win and succeed, no matter what the goal, that they learned in the Teams that gives them their edge.

Another advantage of being in the Teams is the constant training. Schools, both military and civilian, that would be next to impossible to attend, let alone pay for, have active SEALs constantly on the rolls. Many of my Teammates realize that Special Warfare gave them this opportunity and they are thankful for the standing it gave them in life.

Waking up in the morning at five and going out to work is something that I have looked forward to for years. Knowing that I would be working with these guys every day has kept that spring in my step over the years. Being a SEAL has been the one job I have had that has to be experienced to really be understood. The men I have worked with are the best in the world and I would go anywhere, undergo any risk, with them. In most jobs, you work daily with individuals and never really interact with them. In the Teams, when the day's work is over, you stay with your Teammates and they become part of your social life. That makes us an even tighter group.

Even the men I have never had the honor of operating with, those forefathers who stood the test in World War II, Korea, Vietnam, and elsewhere, are Teammates. I have a bond with those men that is closer than many people will ever know in their entire lives. If I am lucky, I will continue to work alongside these men in the future. That is a feeling and a reality that only comes from being a SEAL. And being a SEAL means you have passed through the forge that is Basic Underwater Demolition/SEAL training.

The training regimen has proven itself over time. I hope that the future will not change the standards of training at BUD/S that have proven themselves over and over. The standards have to be maintained, if not raised, to keep the Teams filled with the quality operators it takes to get the job done. And anyone can be a part of the Teams, if they can prove they have the "right stuff." And that is something only the individual himself can determine. The instructors will bring out the very best you have inside of you, but you must first bring that quality with you to training.

In the Teams a nine-to-five routine is almost unknown. Instead, we work until the job is completed. Afterward, when the assignment is completed, come the times that SEAL legends are made of. That is where we learned to say, "When you work hard, you're entitled to play hard."

Throughout my career in Special Warfare, I have been lucky enough to have been at the right place at the right time. Every task that was set before me, I completed and endured. And that just continued to make me stronger. And constantly, I strove to make myself better, to improve my abilities, both physical and mental. That is the only way to be if you are to support your Teammates.

Even with the new technology of war that is astonishing us every day, the Teams will always be needed. A man in the field will always have to be there. And since he is necessary anyway, why not make him the very best available?

Once a Team member, you will remain a Teammate until the day you die. When that day has come and gone, those Teammates who remain will take a moment to remember the ones who went before. The memories of those men who cleared the way, and those who made the ultimate sacrifice, are always in our minds as we strive to remain worthy.

To those individuals out there who want to try the greatest challenge available, who want always to succeed in life, no matter what, the Teams is the place to start down that path.

—Dennis C. Chalker
Command Master Chief Boatswain's Mate,
U.S.N. (Ret.)

# PREFACE

In November 1942, during the North Africa landings, the first U.S. invasion of World War II, seventeen men under the command of a Navy lieutenant drove through rough seas into the mouth of the Sebou River. The mission of those men was to cut a cable blocking access to upriver landing sites. Their first attempt driven back, the men once more went up the Wadi Sebou (Wadi is the Arabic word for river) and blasted through the cable, allowing General Patton's forces to capture a vital airfield.

Identified as a Combat Demolition Unit (CDU), those men returned to the United States and were disbanded. Many of the men from that first CDU reunited in 1943 when a new kind of unit was created, the Navy Combat Demolition Units, or NCDUs. The mission of the NCDUs was simple, and severe. It was intended that they blast a hole through the obstacles defending the beaches of Europe and open the way for the "second front." Though they had no way of knowing it at the time, they were to cut a path for the U.S. forces to follow during the landings at Normandy Beach in June 1944.

Gathered under the command of Lieutenant Commander Draper Kauffmann at the direct command of Admiral Ernest J. King, Chief of Naval Operations, a training center was set up on the grounds of the Naval Amphibious Base at the town of Fort Pierce, on the eastern shore of Florida. Before the new NCDU school was even able to open, the invasion of Sicily was to take place in the Mediterranean. A group of Seabees, civil engineering officers, and other workers experienced with explosives were assembled and further trained in Virginia in May 1943. During the July invasion, these men, now identified as Naval Demolition Unit No.1, conducted operations in support of the Allied forces. After the invasion was over, the men of NDU-1 were sent back to the States. Before the end of the year most of these same men would find themselves at Fort Pierce, training as part of the NCDUs.

NCDU units were set up as groups of five enlisted men under a single officer. The individual NCDUs would each operate seven-man rubber boats, the space for the seventh man in the boat being filled with explosives and equipment. Concentrated classes in the use of explosives were a major part of the NCDU training, but the most knowledgeable men in the world would be of no use if they could not reach the target.

Kauffmann approached the Navy Scouts and Raiders School at Fort Pierce to study what was the first training of its kind to include an organized PT (physical training) program. The pace of the Scouts and Raiders School was too slow to meet the press of coming events faced by Kauffmann and the NCDUs, so Kauffmann had the eight-week course condensed down to one, almost unbelievable, week.

The theory developed by the Scouts and Raiders and adopted and taken further by Draper Kauffmann was that the motivated individual was capable of ten times the physical output he had originally thought possible. That theory was proven to the men who faced it during the six-day period known as Motivation Week, immediately and ever after called Hell Week by all who faced it.

The running, swimming, marches, log PT, and other tasks, or "evolutions" as they were known, drove the men of the NCDU school to the limits of their endurance and beyond. Lack of sleep, constant harassment, impossible objectives that had to be met, and constant physical output brought the men of the NCDUs as close as could be simulated to the mental and physical conditions of an active battlefield. Quitting the grueling training was easy, and many of the men took advantage of this. Forty percent of the men who started NCDU training never finished it. The men who did knew what they were capable of as few men before them ever had.

Before the men of the NCDU school would face their most momentous task, clearing the way for the invasions at Normandy, events in the Pacific theater were building momentum. Admiral Richmond Kelly Turner had seen the horrible losses suffered among the U.S. forces during the invasion at Tarawa in November 1943. The majority of men killed were drowned long before they ever reached the beaches. To prevent a situation like Tarawa repeating itself, Admiral Turner ordered

the creation of new amphibious reconnaissance/ beach obstacle demolition units. These units were to be the Underwater Demolition Teams.

Graduates from the NCDU school at Fort Pierce were awaiting orders while stationed in Hawaii. They had been sent to the Pacific theater to join in operations against the Japanese forces. Taken to be the nucleus of the new units, the men of the NCDUs formed UDTs One and Two. The men of the new UDTs proved their worth during the invasions of the Marshall Islands. Now more UDTs were to be commissioned and sent to further operations in the Pacific.

As the UDTs built up a reputation in the Pacific, the NCDUs faced their task on Omaha and Utah beaches in Normandy on June 6, 1944. Losses were heavy, 30 percent on Utah and 60 to 70 percent on the bloody beaches of Omaha. But the men of the NCDUs blew open breaches in Hitler's Atlantic Wall that allowed the thousands of Allied forces to begin the final assault on the Third Reich. After further operations in southern France the men of the NCDUs moved on to the Pacific to enlarge the UDTs.

The physical demands put on the men while at Fort Pierce had paid off on the sands of Normandy and again on the Pacific islands. Now the men of the UDTs would swim in to enemy beaches days, and sometimes hours, prior to an invasion. Plotting the location of obstacles to incoming landing craft, the UDTs would swim back to those same obstacles during later missions and demolish them with explosives. UDT Eleven performed the Herculean task of mapping 1,300 yards of beaches at Iwo Jima, and then returning and destroying 1,400 obstacles, all of this done in two days of nonstop operations.

Underwater swimming using just the capacity of one's lungs to stay down was developed almost to an art by the World War II UDTs. One-hundred-fifty-pound explosive charges that had to be towed behind a swimmer were used as a matter of course. And the constant barrage of noise, explosions, and gunfire faced by the World War II UDTs were remembered by the later trainees who faced their simulation in So Solly Day, traditionally the last day of Hell Week.

After World War II the UDTs greatly improved their underwater abilities. Cold-water-protection gear and underwater breathing equipment was all tested and adopted. But the freezing waters off Okinawa and Iwo Jima were never forgotten. Trainees still had to face the strength-sapping cold during Underwater Demolition Team Replacement training (UDTR later BUD/S). The best equipment in the world does no good if it is unavailable when needed, but missions still have to be performed, as they were by the near-naked warriors of World War II.

The Korean conflict saw the UDTs operating on dry land as commandos on inland demolition operations. The ability to move from and return to the water made the UDTs easily able to attack vital enemy sites, well behind the normal fighting lines. Operations to infiltrate and exfiltrate guerrillas behind enemy lines were conducted by the UDTs in Korea as well as standard UDT operations in support of the legendary amphibious landing at Inchon.

After the Korean conflict, UDTs became involved with the developing U.S. space program. The physically fit UDT operators would undergo stressful tests to determine if man could even survive being launched into space. A problem was presented during the tests when the scientists found that the UDT operators could absorb punishment previously thought lethal, absorb it and ask for more.

From the very first manned space shot, the UDTs were instrumental in recovering every space capsule. When the Mercury, Gemini, and Apollo capsules splashed down, it was the men of the UDTs who jumped into the sea to secure them.

During the 1960s the UDTs performed duties in Vietnam as the U.S. commitment there continued to grow. Thousands of miles of beaches were surveyed and plotted for possible landing sites. Reconnaissance was performed from aboard ship and submarines. As the ground combat role increased for American forces, men of the UDTs moved inland, performing water recons and demolition operations.

The largest combat demolition project in the history of the Navy was conducted by the men of the UDTs on the Plain of Reeds in Southeast Asia. Five and a half miles of canal were blown up with explosives in the latter months of 1969 and into 1970. Connecting two canals with a ditch capable of being used by small watercraft required 230 tons of high explosive in the form of Mark 8 hose. Twenty-five-foot-long explosive charges weighing up to 750 pounds were moved by hand into position.

When the war in Vietnam ended, the UDTs went back to their support of amphibious operations with the regular fleet forces. Finally, in 1983, the last of the UDTs were decommissioned. The men from the last UDTs went on directly into the new SEAL Teams and SDV (SEAL Delivery Vehicle) Teams that were commissioned the day the UDTs ended.

In the early 1960s President John F. Kennedy directed the military forces of the United States to create new units capable of conducting guerrilla and counterguerrilla operations. The Navy looked to the ranks of the UDTs to fill the mission requirement for the new units. On January 1, 1962, SEAL Teams One and Two were commissioned on the West and East coasts, respectively.

The SEALs (for sea, air, and land, the three environments they operate in) went on to create a legendary record of accomplishments. Operations in Greece, Turkey, the Dominican Republic, the Arctic, and elsewhere, all led up to the SEALs ultimate arena, the jungles and swamps of Southeast Asia.

In Vietnam the SEALs quickly became so feared by the Vietcong that they were given the identifier "the men with green faces." At any time during the night or day, a SEAL could rise up out of the shadows and take down a group of VC guerrillas. Capturing high-ranking VC from out of their beds became something of a SEAL trademark. Spectacular raids and silent observations were all part of the SEALs' operations.

Missions where a group of SEALs would have to work their way through hundreds of yards of mudflats were not unknown. While in the middle of these excruciating operations, the SEALs could look back on the mud they crawled through during Hell Week and just continue on. Slipping in through areas that were considered impassable was a common technique for SEAL operations.

Their mission performances netted the SEALs thousands of enemy troops killed or captured. Dozens of medals and awards were given to the men of SEAL Teams One and Two including 3 Medals of Honor, 5 Navy Crosses, 42 Silver Stars, 402 Bronze Stars, and a host of additional decorations, all of this for men who never went out actively seeking awards.

After Vietnam the SEALs continued to train and face new missions. When the threat of international terrorism increased during the 1970s, the U.S. response to that threat also multiplied. By the early 1980s, SEAL Team Six was commissioned with the express intention of battling the terrorist threat with the same determination that

the Vietcong had been fought in Southeast Asia.

Superbly fit, even for SEALs, the men of SEAL Team Six went on to face combat in Grenada, Panama, Haiti, and elsewhere. The men of the other SEAL Teams also distinguished themselves in those same theaters and additionally in Desert Storm, the waters of the Persian Gulf, Somalia, and the northeastern Mediterranean. Those are just a few of the many places the SEALs have operated in. Additional missions have included training foreign forces in SEAL techniques, supporting the allies of the United States throughout the world, and continuing in an ongoing program of research and development.

To test the U.S. Navy's own security, men from SEAL Team Six were placed in a very new and secret unit known as Red Cell. The men of Red Cell took the part of terrorists themselves. Secure military installations quickly learned what they could expect from a real terrorist attack when Red Cell demonstrated where the weak points were in a security system.

The SEALs constantly push the envelope of endurance and ability. What seems impossible is simply what hasn't been done yet by the men of the Teams. As was almost inevitable, a SEAL has even been in space, having qualified for and served on several space shuttle missions.

# FOREWORD

For those of you who dare to walk with the best or simply have an insatiable desire to find yourselves, this book is a must.

It has been my good fortune to have been a "Team guy," one of the driven few who have navigated the inconceivably difficult challenge of UDTR, now BUD/S, training and, often the harder to achieve, Teammate acceptance. The former is obtainable by anyone driven to the point of near frenzy, the latter only through silent, professional pride.

My class, UDTR Class 29, was the winter class of 1963 conducted at the U.S. Naval Amphibious base, Little Creek, Virginia. To this day this special place is still my home. The memories of Team life prior to, during, and after Vietnam deployment are as fresh today as they were then. It is with the greatest sincerity that I say there can be no honor greater than to have been associated with and accepted by the officers and men of the UDT/SEAL community.

Master Chief Dennis Chalker is truly one of the silent proud who exemplifies the very essence of a true Teammate. His dedication to fel-

low shipmates has been the hallmark of his career. Known as a shooter, he has participated in most actions, overt and covert, since the Vietnam period. After a hitch with the Army 82nd Airborne Division, where he learned how to read, he left the Army and joined the Navy for BUD/S training in Coronado, California. Upon completion of training, he was assigned to SEAL Team One, where he was immediately recruited by a Team brother, Dick Marcinko, as one of the plank owners of SEAL Team Six, starting a long, distinguished naval career in counterterrorism. His final, and most rewarding, tour of duty was with the officers and men, instructors and students, of the "School House" or Naval Special Warfare Training Center. As Command Master Chief under Skipper, Captain Joe Yarborough, he was able to inject the "Operator's" point of view into the training program—the very roots of NAVSPECWAR.

Having seen hundreds of BUD/S students either DOR—drop on request—or graduate, he observed the difference between the unprepared and prepared BUD/S trainee. It is because of his continuing desire to help the Teams and his Teammates that he has written this book with Kevin Dockery to help the aspiring trainee negotiate the physical aspects of training.

Last, but certainly not least, it must be noted that physical ability alone will not get you through training, although it makes for easier sailing. The brain drives desire; without it there is no chance in hell of success in this program. Just remember, gentlemen, it is a case of mind over matter—if you don't mind, it doesn't matter. Hooooyaaaaa!

—HARRY J. HUMPHRIES
UDT22 and SEAL Team Two
Fraternal Order UDT/SEAL—Life member
UDT-SEAL Museum Association—Life member

# ACKNOWLEDGMENTS

TECHNICAL CONSULTANT AND DEMONSTRATOR:
Deverick T. Lampley, Bodies Plus Training Center

DEMONSTRATORS:
Thomas Ferrarie
William Humphries

PHOTOGRAPHER:
Carin A. Baer

ASSISTANT PHOTOGRAPHER:
Lori Carr

HAIR STYLIST:
Anthony Camacho

MAKEUP:
Bonnie Subnick

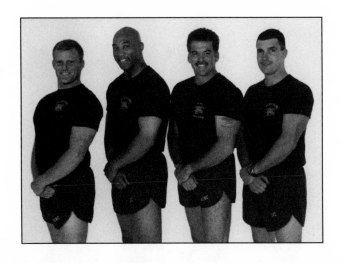

# CONTENTS

# INTRODUCTION

Strongly brought forward to the public's attention only within the last ten years or so, the U.S. Navy SEALs have been one of the least publicized and most secretive of the U.S. military's Special Operations forces. With the publication of a quantity of popular books and the release of a number of movies, the reputation of the Navy SEALs has become widespread. This publicity, not particularly welcomed by the Navy Special Warfare community, along with a general increase in the importance of Special Operations units, has resulted in the raising of the number of recruits volunteering for SEAL training to high levels.

Volunteering to be a SEAL and passing the introductory training are two very widely separated steps. BUD/S, Basic Underwater Demolition/SEAL training, Navy course A-431-0024, is considered by many to be among the most physically demanding training offered in the U.S. military. BUD/S is where the heart and soul of a SEAL is forged and is the most obvious binding factor among SEALs that can be seen by an outsider. For the balance of his life a SEAL will always be able to be identified as a member of a BUD/S class.

That simple number secures him a place in one of the most elite units of fighting men.

At one time BUD/S was offered at two locations, Little Creek, Virginia, and Coronado, California. Since the early 1970s all of the basic SEAL training has been centered in one place, the Naval Special Warfare Training Detachment at the Naval Special Warfare Center, Coronado, California. Developed from the earlier Underwater Demolition Team Replacement (UDTR) training course, BUD/S will give the prospective SEAL a solid base of skills to build his Special Warfare career on. But those skills are hard-won.

For twenty-five weeks trainees will work harder and longer than they ever have before. Even after graduating BUD/S there is still a six-month probationary period before an individual can wear the Naval Special Warfare Insignia that proclaims him a SEAL to anyone who sees it. Only a very few men can face such a long period of intense effort without flagging; most will quit along the way.

Navy Special Warfare is a fully voluntary field. You are not assigned to be a Navy SEAL; you vol-

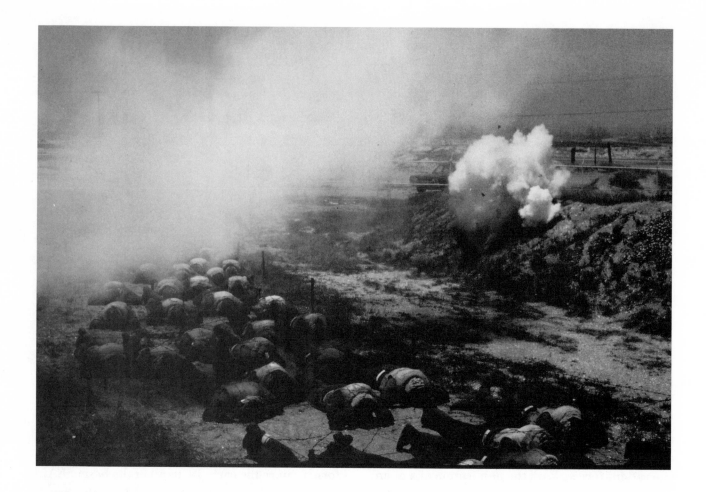

unteer. And you leave by simply quitting. Just by saying, "I quit" or "DOR" (Drop on Request), the training is over. You will be immediately taken out of the class of trainees you were with and be gone from the training center within a short time. It is that ease of quitting that makes BUD/S training so hard.

Prior to arriving at BUD/S, prospective SEALs can attend the Naval Special Warfare BUD/S selection course that is offered at the Naval Training Command at Great Lakes, Illinois. This five-day course introduces the training curriculum, and the physical demands, of BUD/S to prospective volunteers and leaves no question as to what they will be volunteering for.

Once the decision to go to BUD/S has been reached, and the screening test passed, the potential BUD/S student will report to Coronado and be processed in. Prior to beginning formal training, or "classing-up," the student will be assigned to a

group undergoing pretraining. The pretraining period is formally structured into a two-week required course titled BUD/S Indoctrination. It is a time for the student to become more prepared for the physical demands that will be placed on him once he begins BUD/S. Basic exercises, swimming, running, and exposure to the obstacle course are all conducted during this course.

Once a group has classed-up, they begin the first of the three phases of BUD/S training. First Phase, the Basic Conditioning Phase, is eight weeks long. Constant emphasis is put on physical conditioning. Running and swimming are constantly increased in terms of distance while time is cut back as speeds increase. But the time spent doing calisthenics is increased. For five weeks the student will be constantly pushed to better himself and learn to operate as part of a team. As a member of a team, the student will face one of the hardest tasks of training, the fifth week, Hell Week.

For over five days, the student will be pushed to his personal breaking point on a regular basis. The week is one of continuous training. Only five hours of sleep is scheduled for the entire week; exposure to the cold and seemingly impossible tasks will face each man. The physical output will not seem possible, and for many it has not been.

The ease with which the misery of training can end, simply by saying, "I quit," or ringing a brass bell in the middle of the compound, and a student can be warm, dry, and resting, will overwhelm many. It is at this point that the individual must reach down within himself and find that which will keep him going.

Many SEALs and UDT men have talked about going on "automatic" during Hell Week. Not thinking but just continuing for the next moment, and the moment after that. But during BUD/S training you must remain as sharp as possible. Thinking is required. And you have to operate as part of a team or many of the evolutions will be literally impossible. This is the ultimate test of an individual's mental and physical motivation. And there is nothing to compare with the feeling of hearing the order to "secure from Hell Week" and be standing with the very few who made it with you.

The remaining three weeks of First Phase are devoted to learning the various methods of conducting hydrographic surveys, sketching hydrographic charts, and some of the most basic beach reconnaissance conducted by the UDTs since their first days in the Pacific.

It is not enough to simply complete First Phase and continue with training. The physical fitness standards required to pass First Phase are as follows:

| | |
|---|---|
| 50-meter underwater swim | Pass/fail |
| Drownproofing test | Pass/fail |
| Basic lifesaving test | Pass/fail |
| 1/2-mile pool swim without fins | Completion |
| 3/4-mile pool swim without fins | Completion |
| 1-mile pool swim without fins | 60 minutes |
| 1-mile bay swim without fins | 70 minutes |
| 1-mile bay swim with fins | 50 minutes |
| 1 1/2-mile ocean swim with fins | 95 minutes |
| 2-mile timed run (weekly in boots) | 32 minutes |
| Obstacle Course | 15 minutes |

Once all of these physical standards have been reached, and preferably exceeded, the student moves on to Second Phase.

Second Phase is devoted to diving. Now that the individual has proven to the instructor staff that he has the will to be a SEAL, the in-depth training will commence. During the seven weeks of Second Phase, the student will be taught combat scuba swimming. He will learn to use two types of scuba equipment: the standard open-circuit compressed air system so familiar to sport divers, and

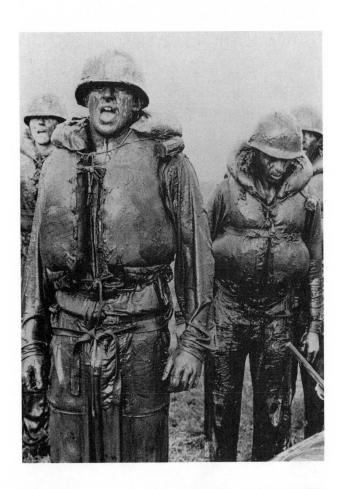

the closed-circuit, 100-percent oxygen system used for most dives in the Teams.

Students will learn how to navigate underwater and transport themselves to a target without detection. Basic combat swimmer techniques will be taught; they are the skills that separate the SEALs from all of the other Special Operations forces in the U.S. military. The students will learn that the SEAL is more at home in the hostile environment of the water than in any other place.

While they are in Second Phase, physical training will not be ignored. Greater demands will be made on the students in terms of distances covered in both swims and runs. Four-mile runs, two-mile swims, and the obstacle course must all be completed within shortened time limits. For passing Second Phase, the physical fitness standards are:

| | |
|---|---|
| 2-mile swim with fins | 80 minutes |
| 4-mile timed run (weekly in boots) | 31 minutes |
| Obstacle course | 11 minutes |
| 5½-mile ocean swim with fins | Completed |

Third Phase is the land warfare and demolitions phase of SEAL training. During the ten weeks of Third Phase, the first four weeks are spent both in a classroom environment and in the open air studying the skills of modern warfare. Land navigation, rappelling, small-unit tactics, patrolling techniques, infantry tactics, military explosives, and demolitions are all taught in detail. The last five weeks of Third Phase are spent on San Clemente Island, practicing the skills learned earlier in a practical environment.

Additional training will be given in modern arms. All of the small arms a SEAL can expect to work with on a regular basis will be studied, learned, and practiced. Live firing with both small arms and explosives will be conducted. And the physical training will continue. Distances will be increased and minimum times lowered. The minimum physical standards to pass Third Phase are:

| | |
|---|---|
| 2-mile ocean swim with fins | 75 minutes |
| 4-mile timed run | 30 minutes |
| Obstacle course | 10 minutes |

Academic standards will also be high throughout BUD/S. A SEAL is an intelligent, thinking man, not an overmuscled, drilled machine. The standards for the written tests are a score of 80 percent or better for officers and 70 percent or better for enlisted men.

The officers in the SEALs are a unique breed. In no other training course in the Navy are officers driven as hard as at BUD/S. They are not only expected to complete the course; they are expected to lead their men while doing it. A SEAL officer has completed every evolution and event that any other SEAL who graduated BUD/S has. If anything, the instructors are harder on the officers because they may have to follow that same officer later in their Special Warfare career.

But the graduation from BUD/S, for both officer and enlisted man, is a reinforcement that they have done something very few men have done before them. After graduation three weeks will be spent at the Army Airborne School in Fort Benning, Georgia. BUD/S graduates will learn basic parachuting and earn their jump wings before continuing on to their initial assignment in the Teams.

Assignments to an active SEAL or SEAL Delivery Vehicle (SDV) Team follow graduation from jump school. For the next six months the new graduates will undergo a probationary period. After successfully completing their probation the new SEALs will be awarded the SEAL classification code and their Naval Special Warfare Insignia, the Trident.

# WARM-UPS AND COOL-DOWNS

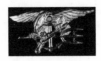

**During training you had to constantly improve,
to beat your best time, or you would be out.**
**—SEAL, Class 15**

A WARM-UP ROUTINE should be considered an essential part of any workout routine. This is especially important prior to conducting a strenuous period of exercise such as the Schedule III program.

A good warm-up raises the heart rate of the exerciser, increasing the flow of blood to the muscles. The increased blood flow raises the temperature of the muscles as well as makes a large amount of nutrients and oxygen available to them prior to heavy work. An additional benefit of a warm-up is an increase in the elasticity of the muscles, ligaments, and tendons of the body, making them more flexible and better prepared for work.

Present evidence indicates that a warm-up not only increases overall performance of an exercise routine; it also lowers the risk of injury. Warming up prior to an intense workout may also lower the risk of injury to the heart itself.

A general warm-up routine involves large-muscle exercises rather than specific concentration on a smaller muscle group. For a calisthenic workout, jumping jacks, arm rotations, and other exercises are used.

Prior to conducting a heavy-lift exercise with either free weights or a machine, it is suggested that a specific warm-up be done first with at least a 50 percent lighter weight. An example would be if a person is planning to complete 3 sets of 12 reps of 200-pound bench presses, he would first warm up with a single set of 10 reps with a 100-pound or less weight.

An additional part of a warm-up routine should include a set of stretches. Stretching adds to the overall flexibility of the muscles and tendons prior to conducting an exercise. The stretches would be done after the warm-up calisthenics. The same set of stretches listed for the postworkout cool-down can be added to the warm-up routine.

## WARM-UP EXERCISES

❑

**ARM ROTATIONS**
**JUMPING JACKS**
**HALF JUMPING JACKS**

❑

### ARM ROTATIONS

**Muscle groups.** Shoulders and upper chest, especially the deltoid and pectoral muscles.

This warm-up loosens up the shoulders, chest, and arm muscles and is especially valuable prior to an upper-body workout.

### Technique

1. Stand up with the feet shoulder-width apart and the arms extended straight out from the shoulders. Clench the fists lightly and slowly circle the arms in a clockwise (forward) direction, making small circular motions with the circle about 8 to 10 inches in diameter. Each rotation should take about one second to complete.

Enlarge the rotations gradually through the clockwise set making circular motions several feet in diameter.

Gradually reduce the size of the rotations until you are back to making circles 8 to 10 inches in diameter.

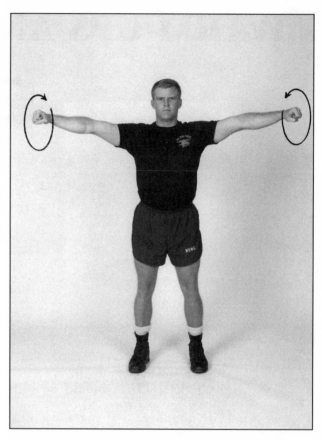

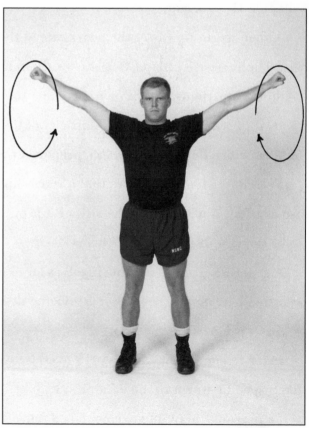

2. Reverse the direction of the arm rotations, circling the hands in a counterclockwise (aft) direction. Continue through the same number of rotations as before: doing the small, then large, and then back to small rotations.

3. Turn the arms forward, straight out from the chest, without letting them drop. Continue with clockwise (outboard) rotations doing the same number of small circles before rotating the arms in larger circles and then back to small.

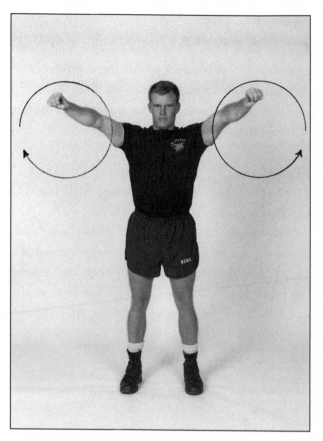

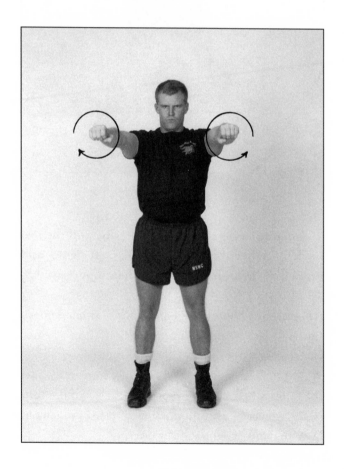

4. Staying in the same position, reverse the direction of the hands, rotating them in a counterclockwise (inboard) direction. Make the same-sized small circular motions with the fists, expanding into large circles, and then back to small.

**Repetition.** This exercise is counted by the number of rotations in a given direction.

## JUMPING JACKS

**Muscle groups.** Legs, hips, shoulders, and chest, especially the deltoid muscle of the shoulders and the gastrocnemius muscle of the calf.

This exercise moves the entire body, giving one of the better overall warm-up effects.

### Technique

1. Start in the standing position, with the feet together and the arms flat at the sides. Jumping lightly into the air, spread the feet beyond shoulder-width apart while simultaneously raising the arms above the head. The hands cross one behind the other above the head at the same time as the feet land back on the ground in the spread position. (Count 1)

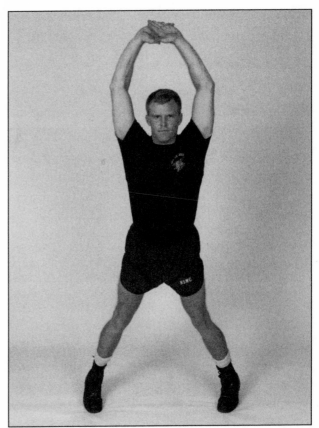

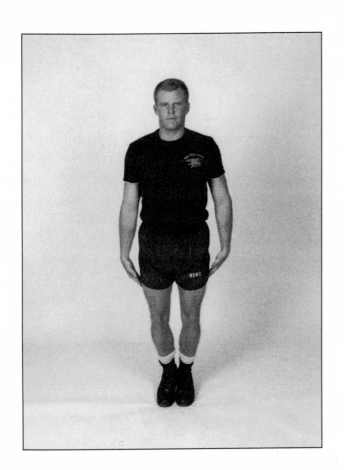

2. Again jumping slightly into the air, pull the feet back together, keeping the legs straight, and pulling the arms back down to the sides. (Count 2)

**Repetition.** The above completes a single repetition of a two-count jumping jack.

WARNINGS. Do not allow the hands to slap against the sides when coming down on the second count of the exercise. Maintain a coordinated movement over the entire range of the exercise.

## HALF JUMPING JACKS

**Muscle Groups.** Legs, hips, shoulders, and chest, especially the deltoid muscle of the shoulders, the pectoralis major muscle of the chest, and the gastrocnemius muscle of the calf.

This exercise moves the entire body, giving one of the better overall warm-up effects with a concentration of work in the shoulders and chest.

### Technique

1. Start in the standing position, with the feet together and the arms flat at the sides. Jumping lightly into the air, spread the feet beyond shoulder-width apart while simultaneously raising the arms level with the shoulders. Stop the upward movement of the arms as they come level with the shoulders at the same time as the feet land back on the ground in the spread position. (Count 1)

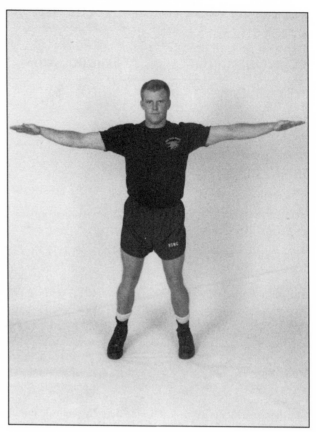

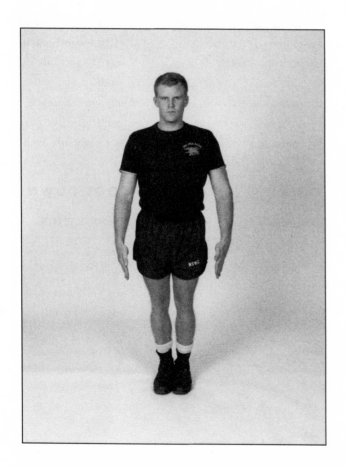

2. Again jumping slightly into the air, pull the feet back together, keeping the legs straight, and pulling the arms back down to the sides. (Count 2)

**Repetition.** The above completes a single repetition of a two-count half jumping jack.

WARNINGS. Do not allow the hands to slap against the sides when coming down on the second count of the exercise. Maintain a coordinated movement over the entire range of the exercise while not allowing the arms to move above the shoulders.

## WARM-UP WORKOUTS INCLUDING STRETCHES

| EXERCISE/STRETCH | REPS/DURATION |
| --- | --- |
| Jumping jacks | 25 |
| Half jumping jacks | 15 |
| Arm rotations | 15 each fore/aft |
| Press, press, fling | 10 |
| Hi Jack/Hi Jill | 10 |
| Up, back, and over | 10 |
| Triceps stretch | 2 sets, 15 seconds each |
| Trunk side stretch | 2 sets, 15 seconds each |
| Standing hamstring stretch | 2 at 15 seconds each |
| Swimmer stretch | 2 at 15 seconds each |
| Quadriceps stretch | 2 sets, 15 seconds each |
| Rhomboid stretch | 2 sets, 15 seconds each |
| Lower-back stretch | 2 at 15 seconds each |

## RUNNING (SWIMMING) STRETCHES

This set of warmup and loosening stretches should be performed prior to and after each run or swim, whether distance or interval.

| STRETCH | REPS/DURATION |
| --- | --- |
| Hurdler stretch | 4 sets, 15 seconds each |
| Groin stretch | 4 at 15 seconds each |
| Calf/Achilles stretch | 4 sets, 15 seconds each |
| Sitting calf/hamstring stretch | 4 at 15 seconds each |

Additional beneficial stretching can be done during a weight training session. After each exercise, perform two of the stretches that affect the primary muscles targeted by the movement. Hold each stretch for fifteen seconds.

## COOL-DOWNS

A cool-down helps lower muscle temperatures and metabolic rates back to normal levels. It also helps prevent or cut down on stiffness and soreness that may develop later and in general helps the body recover from sustained physical activity. The period of time a cool-down takes also helps prevent cramping and heart difficulties, which can take place if a shower is taken too soon after a workout.

## COOL-DOWN

| STRETCH | REPS/DURATION |
| --- | --- |
| Triceps stretch | 2 sets, 15 seconds each |
| Trunk side stretch | 2 sets, 15 seconds each |
| Standing hamstring stretch | 2 at 15 seconds each |
| Swimmer stretch | 2 at 15 seconds each |
| Quadriceps stretch | 2 sets, 15 seconds each |
| Rhomboid stretch | 2 sets, 15 seconds each |
| Lower back stretch | 2 at 15 seconds each |

## RUNNING (SWIMMING) COOL-DOWN

| STRETCH | REPS/DURATION |
| --- | --- |
| Hurdler stretch | 4 sets, 15 seconds each |
| Groin stretch | 4 at 15 seconds each |
| Calf/Achilles stretch | 4 sets, 15 seconds each |
| Sitting calf/hamstring stretch | 4 at 15 seconds each |

# STRETCHING

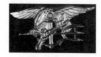

**The harder they made it for us, the harder I worked.**

**I was in the SEAL class because UDT was what**

**I wanted and they weren't going to make me stop unless**

**I died or just came apart along the way.**

**—SEAL, Class 27**

PROPERLY DONE STRETCHES are an important part of a balanced physical fitness program. Done as a warm-up routine, as an exercise program in themselves on off-days, and as part of a calisthenics program, stretches benefit the body in several ways. The stretching routine, which works all of the body's major muscle groups, increases the blood flow to the muscles while loosening them up and increasing flexibility. The increase in flexibility aids greatly in reducing the chance of injury or causing lower-back pain while exercising. The increase in blood flow aids the muscles in receiving nutrients and oxygen during a workout and helps remove waste products more efficiently. A stretch routine is also a major part of the cool-down needed after a workout. The after-workout stretch also helps prevent muscular stiffness and pain.

Stretches are primarily done statically; you stretch and hold the position. And you stretch to the point of discomfort, but not of pain. A tightness will be felt in the muscles and tendons affected by the movement as the stretch is extended. Pull into this tightness but do not extend beyond it. As the workouts continue, the tightness will gradually be harder and harder to reach as the muscles and joints gain flexibility. Never bounce or move hard against the stretch to push the muscles. This action can cause serious injury by forcing the muscles past their maximum stretch. As a rule, stretches are done as a slow, controlled movement while continuing to breathe normally. The actions of a stretch are increased by extending the movement and the time spent in the stretch. Most stretches are initially done for 15-second periods. This time can be gradually extended until 30 to 45 seconds are spent in each repetition of a stretch.

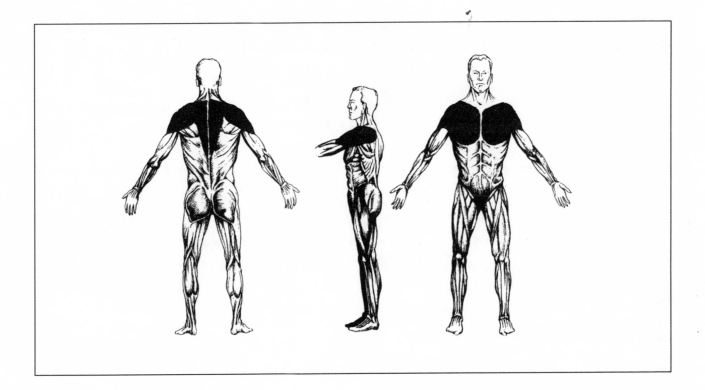

## HI JACK/HI JILL

**Muscle groups.** Shoulders and upper chest and back, particularly the deltoids, pectoralis major, and trapezius.

This is an active stretch combining motion and pull. The action is done at a good pace and part of the stretch is from the muscles acting to stop the movement of the arms.

### Technique

1. From a standing position with the feet about shoulder-width apart, extend the right arm out above the shoulder, angling slightly above the shoulder line, with the elbow bent at a 90-degree angle. The left arm is down at the left side with the elbow bent the same as the right and extending out far enough for the hand to be able to pass by the leg.

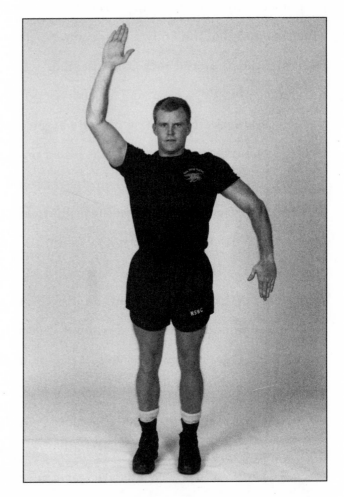

2. The right hand is rotated back from the shoulder with some force and stopped when it has traveled about 6 to 10 inches. The left hand is also forcefully moved to the rear 6 to 10 inches, in concert with the right hand, and stopped. All rotations are taking place in the shoulders with the upper and lower arms staying in line with each other. (Count 1)

3. The right and left arms are moved back into their original position and the backward movement repeated. (Count 2)

4. The position of the arms is switched. The right arm is now down along the right leg and the left arm is raised above the shoulder. Six- to 10-inch rearward movements of both arms are done and stopped. (Count 3)

5. The arms are moved back to the forward position and forceful rear movement repeated. (Count 4)

**Repetition.** The above completes one repetition of a Hi Jack/Hi Jill stretch.

**Advantages.** This dynamic motion helps stretch and warm up the muscles with both the movement and the sudden stopping of the movement. The action must be done with some snap for maximum effect.

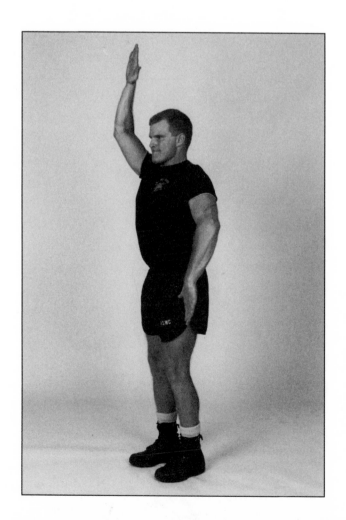

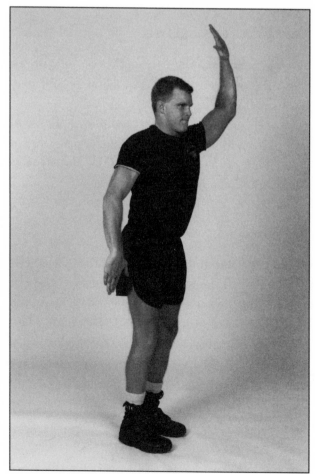

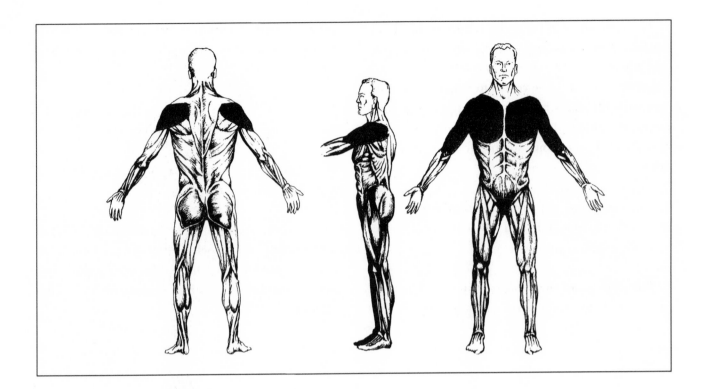

## PRESS, PRESS, FLING

**Muscle groups.** Arms, shoulders, and upper chest, particularly the biceps, deltoids, and pectoralis major.

This is an active stretch combining motion and pull. The action is done at a good pace and a major part of the stretch is from the muscles acting to stop the movement of the arms.

### Technique

1. From the standing position, with the feet spaced shoulder-width apart, raise the arms so that the upper arms are even with the shoulders. Bend the forearms inward with the hands in fists, palms facing down. The arms are bent so that the knuckles of the fists lightly touch in front of the upper chest. The eyes remain looking forward.

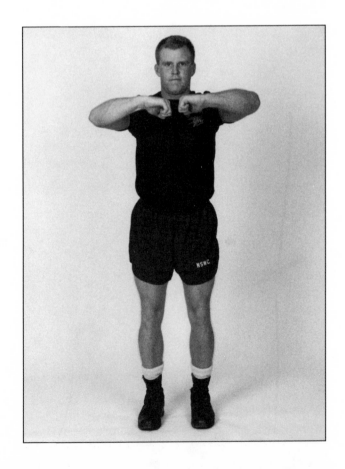

2. With the arms still bent, swing the elbows to the rear until the knuckles of the hands are facing forward. (Count 1—press)

3. Bring the arms forward to the starting position, and the rear press movement is repeated. (Count 2—press)

4. The arms are brought forward again to the starting position. Then swing them back with the elbows opening as the arms move to the rear. Open the hands as the arms move. Preferably level with the shoulders, the arms move straight out past the sides with the hands open and the palms facing forward. As the arms reach their maximum backward swing, they are forced back slightly to stretch the chest muscles. (Count 3—fling)

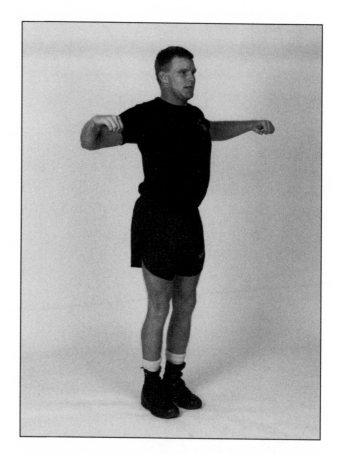

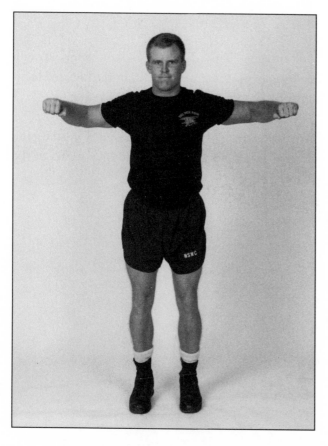

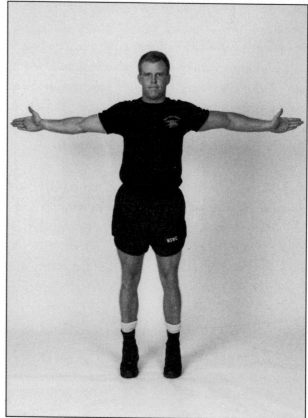

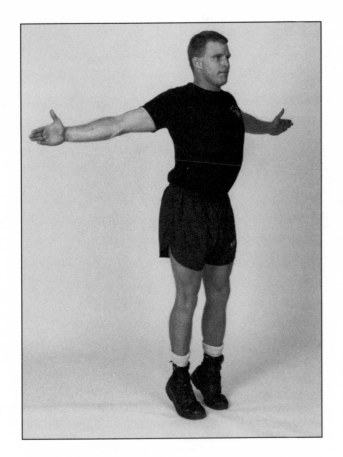
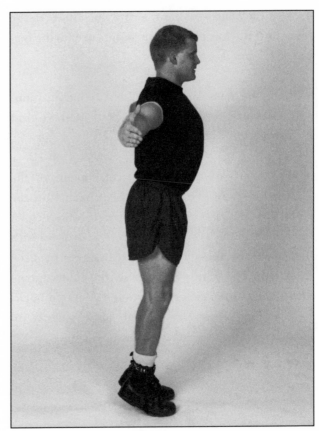

5. The arms are swung forward again, bending in at the elbows as they move with the hands closing into fists. The swing ends with the arms back in the starting position, bent in front of the chest, level with the shoulders and the knuckles of the fists facing each other, palms down.

**Repetition.** The above completes one repetition of a three-count press, press, fling stretch.

**Advantages.** This dynamic motion helps stretch and warm up the muscles with both the movement and the sudden stopping of the movement.

WARNINGS. Do not force the arms back hard on the fling (Count 3) as this can strain the muscles of the chest.

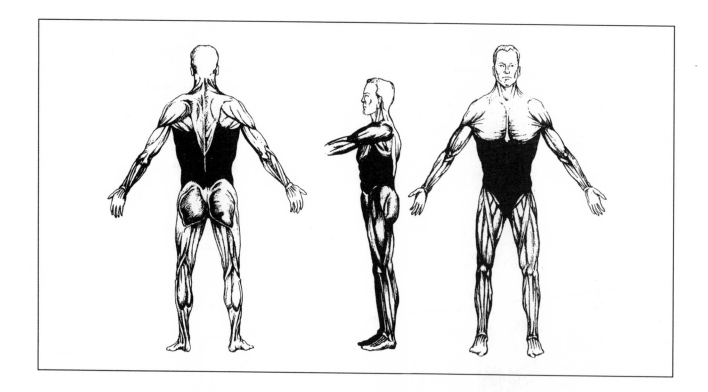

## SIDE BENDERS

**Muscle groups.** Trunk and abdomen, especially the internal and external obliques, rectus abdominis, and to a lesser extent, the latissimus dorsi.

This exercise stretches and works most of the major muscle groups of the upper body and trunk, at the same time including the shoulders and arms.

### Technique

1. Start in the standing position, the feet spread greater than shoulder-width apart. The hands rest lightly on the hips with the elbows bent and out to the sides.

2. Taking the right hand from the hip, slide the hand and arm down the outside of the right leg. Raise the left arm above the shoulder, bending the arm at the elbow so that the wrist rests on top of the head. The hand is open and the palm facing forward. Alternatively, the right arm can be extended straight up above the shoulder at the individual's discretion. Maintain the same arm

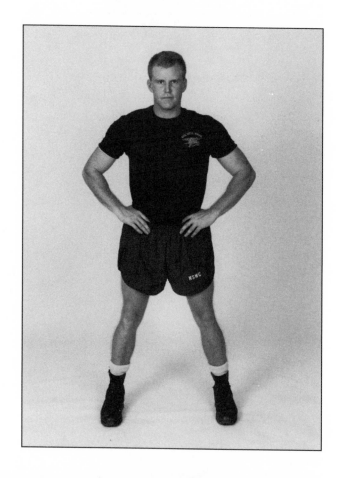

position throughout both parts (sides) of the movement. Tilt the body to the right side as far as it will go while keeping the legs and back in the same plane. Hold the tilted position for two seconds. (Count 1)

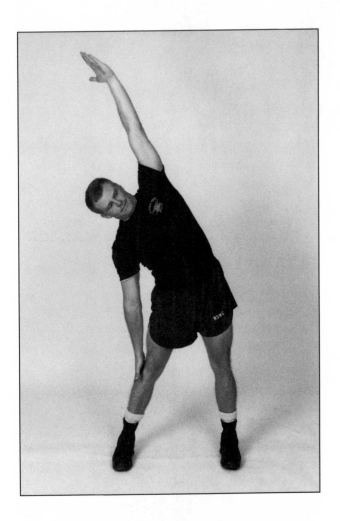

3. Return to the upright position slowly and smoothly and switch arms. Extend the left arm down beside the left leg and extend the right arm above the shoulder. Tilt the body to the left as far as it will go and hold the position for two seconds. (Count 2)

4. Return to the upright position in a slow, smooth movement.

**Repetition.** The above completes a single repetition of a two-count side bender.

WARNINGS. Breathe out during the stretch portion of the exercise and do not bounce to the side.

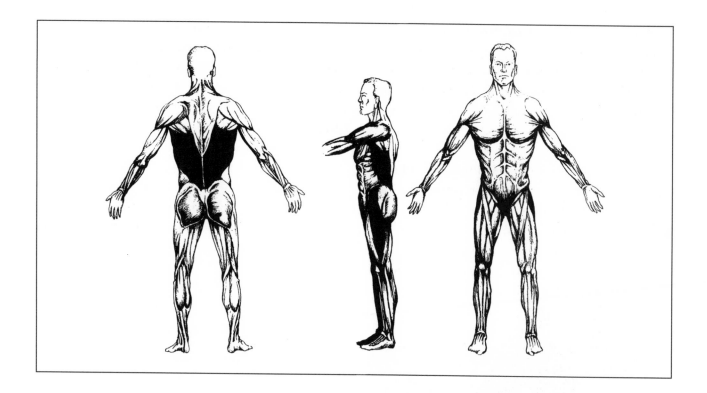

## LOWER-BACK STRETCH (SPINAL TWIST)

**Muscle groups.** The lower back and outside of the thigh, particularly the latissimus dorsi, lumbodorsal fascia, sacrospinalis, and vastus laturalis.

This stretch concentrates on the lower back, one side at a time, as well as the outside muscles of the thigh. The muscles of the upper back, hips, and rib cage also receive some benefit from the movement.

### Technique

1. In the upright sitting position with the legs extended straight out, bring the right knee up, bending the leg, and cross the right foot over to rest on the outside of the left knee. Flexing the right leg, press the knee down toward the floor as much as possible. Extend both arms straight out from the shoulders, hands flat and palms down toward the floor. The head remains upright, facing out between the hands. Hold the back as straight upright as possible.

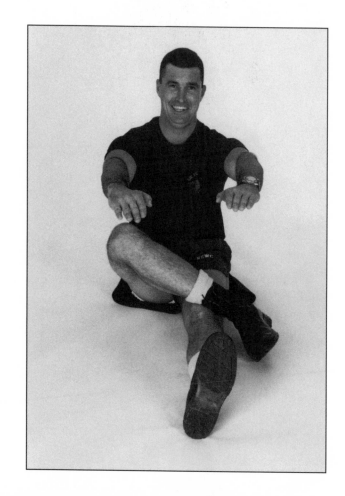

2. While keeping the arms straight out, twist the body to the right, keeping the head looking out between the hands. Turn the body to its maximum extent. Breathe normally and hold the stretch for 15 seconds. Later, you can hold the stretch for 30 seconds as flexibility increases.

3. Return to the facing-forward position. Change legs, crossing the left foot to rest against the outside of the right knee. Extend the arms out straight from the shoulders.

4. Twist the body to the left with the arms extended and the head looking out between the hands. Turn the body to its maximum extent. Breathe normally and hold the stretch for fifteen seconds. Hold the stretch for thirty seconds as flexibility increases.

**Repetition.** The above completes one full movement of the lower back stretch.

WARNINGS. Do not hold your breath during the stretch. Push back with the arm only to hold the bent leg stationary, not to force the twist. Do not bounce on the twist.

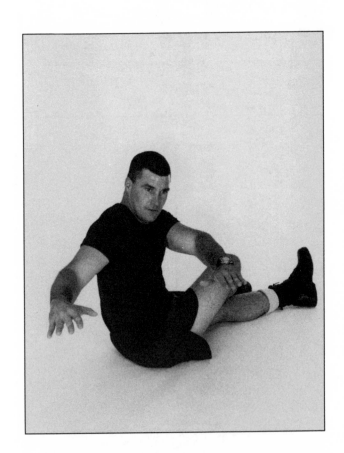

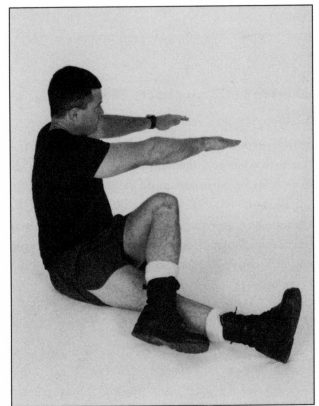

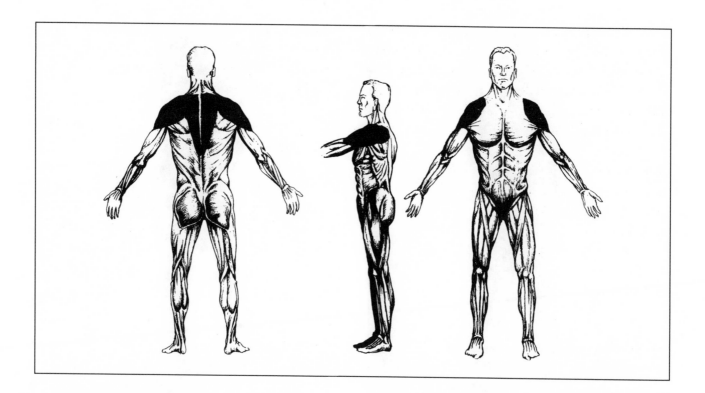

## RHOMBOID STRETCH

**Muscle groups.** Shoulder and upper back, especially the major and minor rhomboid, trapezius, and deltoid muscles.

Pressing one arm with the other allows this movement to stretch the muscles of the shoulder to their maximum extent. The angle of the arm across the throat helps minimize the overstretching of the muscles.

### Technique

1. While standing straight with the head held up, bring the right arm up and across the front of the neck, underneath the chin and bent at the elbow. The right forearm is wrapped around the left side of the neck and extends out over the left shoulder. The upper left arm is held down at the side and the left forearm bent up with the palm of the left hand placed on the outside of the right elbow.

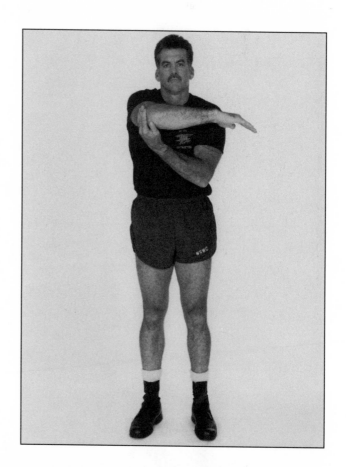

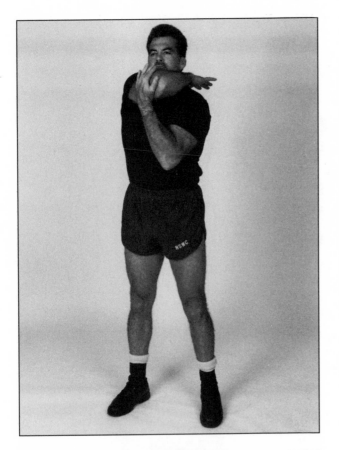

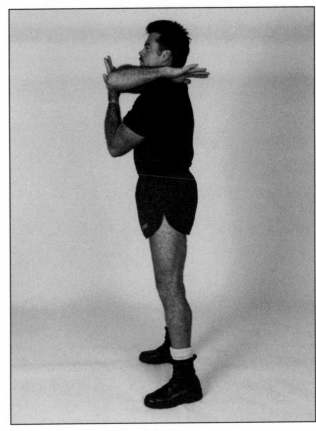

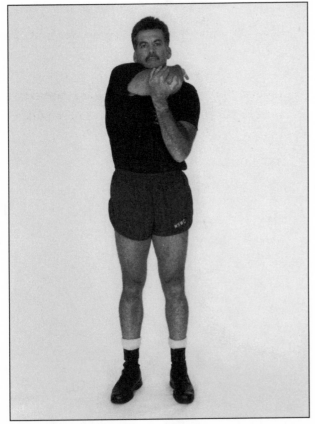

2. The right elbow is pushed in firmly by the left hand, stretching the right shoulder. While breathing normally, hold the stretch for 15 seconds and then relax.

3. The position of the arms is switched with the left arm wrapped underneath the chin and extended out over the right shoulder. The left elbow is pressed in firmly with the palm of the right hand and the stretch held for 15 seconds.

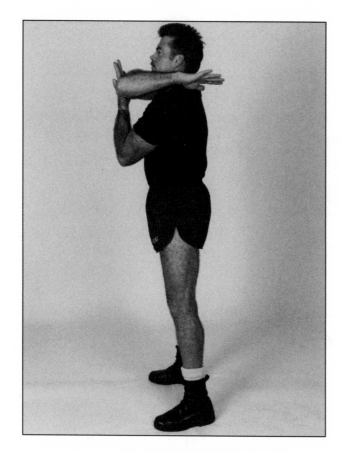 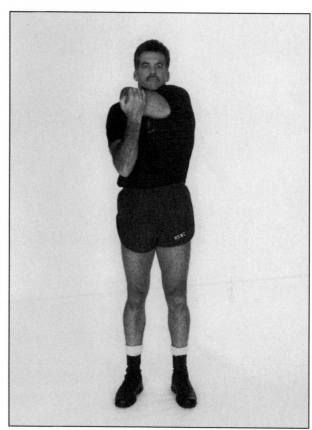

**Repetition.** The above is one repetition of the rhomboid stretch for both arms.

**Advantages.** This movement fully works the shoulder muscles with pressure from the other arm providing the stretch. The location of the arm and neck help prevent overstretching of the shoulder.

WARNINGS. Care must be taken to prevent excess pressure on the throat. The elbow is pressed over the shoulder and not back into the throat.

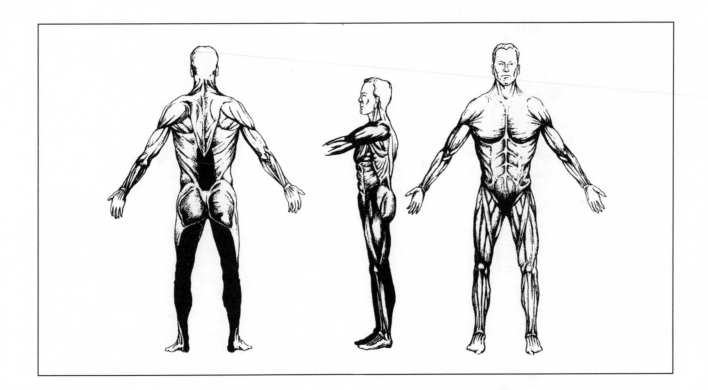

## SITTING HAMSTRING STRETCH

**Muscle groups.** Rear of the thighs, calves, and lower back, specifically the hamstrings, the gastrocnemius, soleus, and plantaris muscles as well as the achilles tendon, and the lumbodorsal fascia and sacrospinalis muscles.

This stretch affects the whole of the back of the leg. If the muscles are tight, the lower back also receives benefit from this movement.

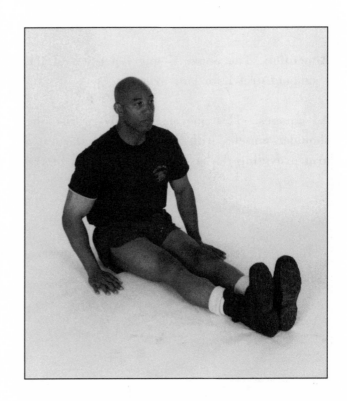

### Technique

1. In the sitting position, extend the legs straight out and hold them together. Hold the feet with the toes pointed up. Put the arms down to the sides, resting the palms on the ground, to get into the proper upright posture and position. Extend the arms out along the tops of the legs, hands flat and palms down toward the tops of the legs.

2. Take a deep breath and bend forward on the slow exhale, extending the hands down toward the toe. Keep the back as straight as possible and the head upright and bend from the hips. Bend forward to the stretch, keeping the legs straight and the toes pointed up. Try to touch the toes with the fingertips. Keep the head upright during the stretch. Hold the bent stretch for 15 seconds and relax.

**Repetition.** The above is one repetition of the sitting hamstring stretch.

**Advantages.** This movement is felt first in the back of the knees and throughout the back of the lower leg. Keeping the toes pointed up increases the stretch for the calf muscles.

**Disadvantages.** This stretch cannot be held for long periods of time as the diaphragm is pressed in by the organs and breathing is difficult.

**Uses.** This stretch is used in place of the standing hamstring stretch when there is nothing available to hold on to for support, or balance cannot otherwise be held.

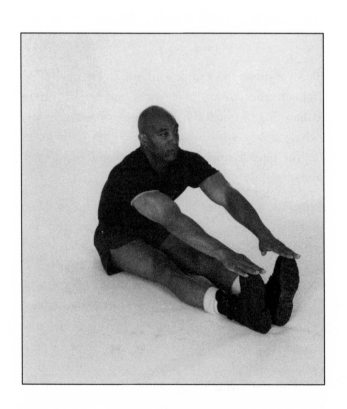

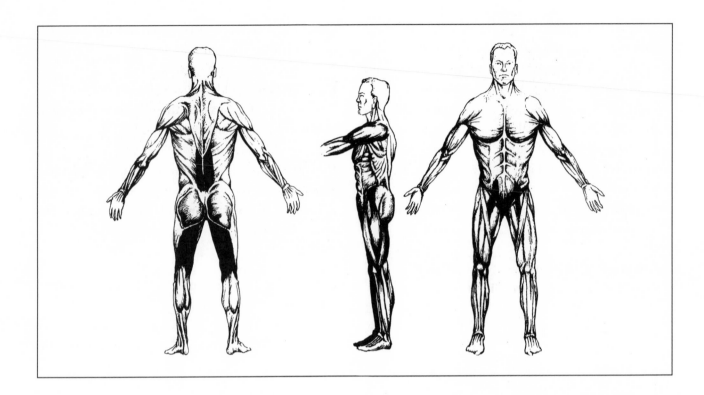

## SITTING HEAD TO KNEES

**Muscle groups.** Back of the thigh, groin, and lower back, especially the hamstrings, psoas major, iliacus, and the lumbodorsal fascia and sacrospinalis.

This movement combines the stretching of the legs and groin with a twisting action of the trunk. It is often used in the martial arts to increase the ability to spread the legs without injury.

### Technique

1. In the sitting position, spread the legs in a V to the maximum extent, stretching the groin tightly but not to the point of pain. The arms are extended out from the shoulders with the elbows bent and the hands lightly cupped behind the ears.

2. After taking a breath, slowly exhale and bend the body down toward the left leg and into the stretch. Bend from the hips and keep the back straight. The hands remain cupped behind the ears while the left elbow touches the left knee. The backs of the knees are kept flat on the floor and the toes pointed up. Hold the stretch for 15 seconds.

3. Straighten the trunk and tilt to the right leg. Repeat the procedure with the right elbow attempting to touch the right knee. Breathe in and exhale slowly, bending into the stretch while keeping the back straight. Hold the stretch for 15 seconds.

*Note.* An additional stretch can be included when in this position. With the legs spread and the trunk facing forward, the arms remain with the hands cupped behind the ears. Bend directly forward, between the legs, with the elbows pointing to their respective knees. A breath is taken and exhaled slowly while bending forward into the stretch. The backs of the knees are kept in contact with the floor, the legs spread, and the toes are pointed straight up. Keep the back straight and try to bend at the hips. Hold the stretch for 15 seconds.

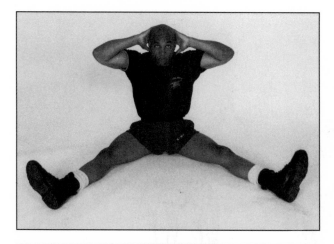

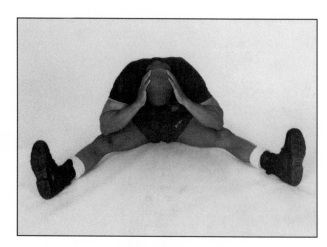

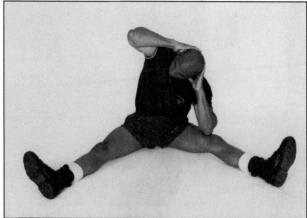

**Repetition.** The above completes one repetition of the head to knee stretch with an additional groin stretch.

**Advantages.** The spread for this stretch can be gradually increased as flexibility improves. Some individuals can spread the legs out straight to the sides, bend flat along the leg, or lay flat on the floor in the optional stretch.

**Disadvantages.** This stretch can pull heavily on the groin.

WARNINGS. Do not bounce during the stretch. Bouncing can cause serious injury by overstretching the muscles of the groin or legs. Keeping the back straight and bending from the hips helps minimize strain on the lower back. Do not pull the head to the side or forward with the hands at any time during the movement.

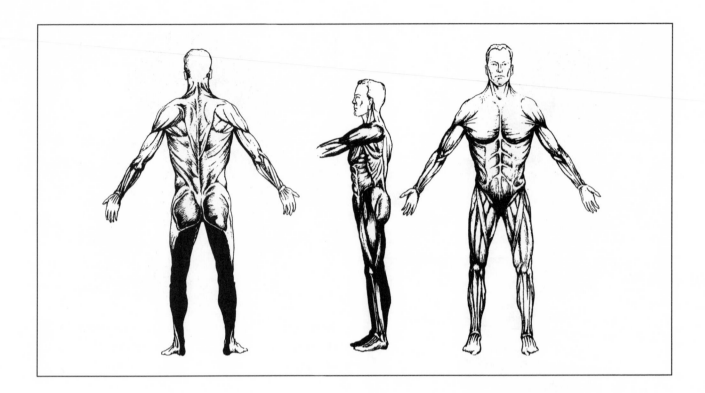

## STANDING HAMSTRING STRETCH

**Muscle groups.** Rear of the thigh and calf, especially the hamstrings, and the gastrocnemius, soleus, and plantaris muscles.

This is a difficult stretch and may require some support to maintain balance.

### Technique

1. From an upright posture with the hands held loosely at the sides, cross the right foot over and in front of the left leg. The feet should be held close together with the lower legs crossed at or above the shins.

2. With the head remaining upright and facing forward, bend from the hips into the stretch. Take a breath and exhale slowly, bending forward into the stretch. Extend the arms out to the floor, touching it if possible to maintain balance. As the stretch progresses, try to place the palms of the hands flat on the floor but do not bounce the body.

Hold the stretch for 15 seconds, breathing normally, and then slowly stand upright.

3. When upright, switch the feet, crossing the left foot over the right.

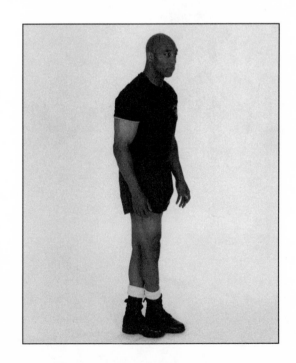

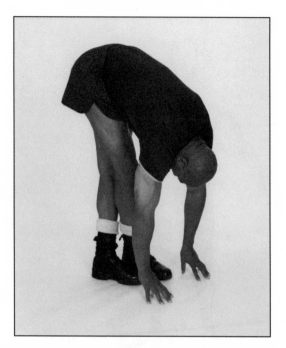

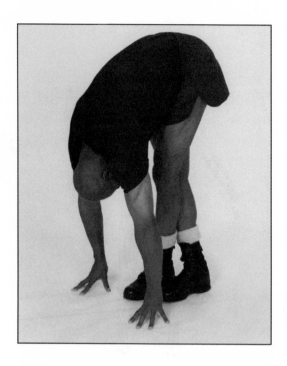

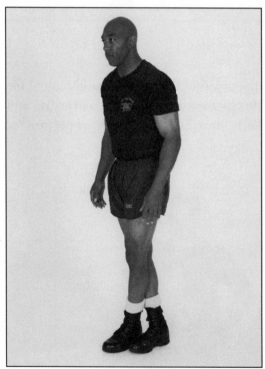

**Repetition.** The above is one full repetition of a standing hamstring stretch.

**Advantages.** This is a relatively easy standing hamstring stretch, especially if support is available.

**Disadvantages.** It is very easy to become dizzy coming out of this stretch. Take care not to lose your balance. Breathing can be difficult while in the stretch as the abdomen and diaphragm are closed in and compressed.

WARNINGS. Breathe normally during the stretch and take care to maintain balance. Do not bounce the body when extending the hands to the floor. Lay the palms flat only when the body has stretched to the point where there is a pull in the backs of the legs and not a pain.

4. Breathe normally and bend forward into the stretch on the exhalation. Place the hands down for support as needed and try to put the palms flat on the floor. While breathing normally, hold the stretch for 15 seconds and then return upright slowly.

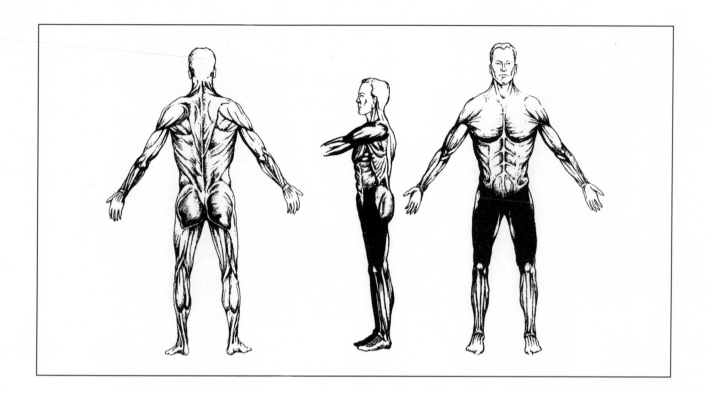

## QUADRICEPS (OUTER THIGH) STRETCH

**Muscle groups.** Front of the thigh, particularly the quadriceps femoris.

This movement stretches the outer thigh while also developing balance and having some beneficial effects on the lower back and abdominals.

### Technique

1. While standing straight, space the feet slightly greater than shoulder-width apart, angling the toes outward. With the elbows pointing down and the upper arms remaining along the sides of the chest, place the palms of the hands together in front of the chest with the fingertips pointed up.

2. Squat down, bending at the knees with the back straight and the head held upright. With the knees bent at about a 90-degree angle or less, place the elbows against the inside of the knees. Push outward on the knees with the elbows for the stretch,

keeping the palms of the hands together. Hold the stretch for 15 seconds, breathing normally, and relax. Slowly straighten to the upright posture.

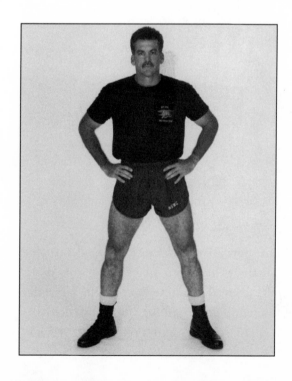

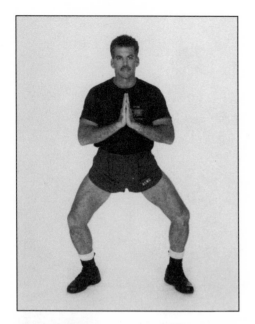

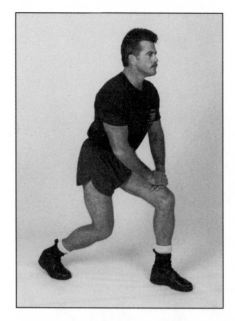

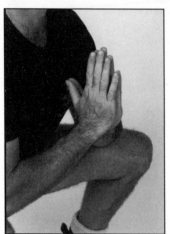

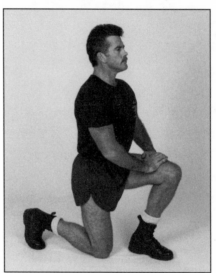

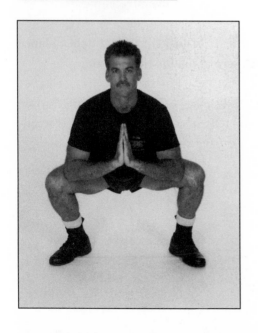

3. From the upright posture with the legs remaining in position, turn to face the left leg, rotating the feet so that the toes point to the left. Squat down, bending the legs at the knees. Bend the left knee at 90 degrees and lower the right knee to four to six inches above the floor. Try to put the heel of the right foot on the floor for the stretch. The hands may be put on the forward knee for balance. Hold the stretch for 15 seconds while breathing normally and then slowly straighten into an upright posture.

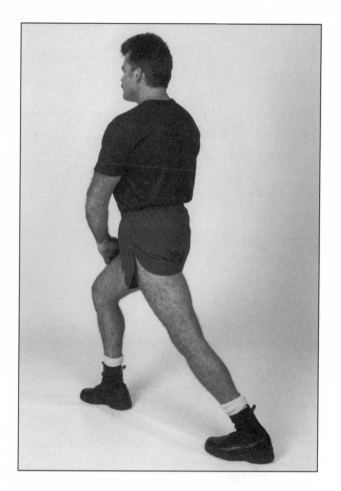

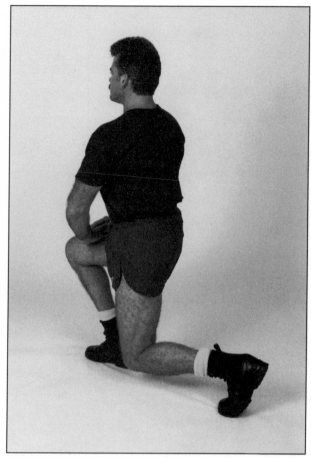

4. Turn and face the right leg, switching directions while pivoting the feet. The right leg is now forward and bends at the knee to 90 degrees. Squat down, bending the legs at the knees. Bend the right knee at 90 degrees and lower the left knee to 4 to 6 inches above the floor. Try to put the heel of the left foot on the floor for the stretch. Put the hands on the forward knee for balance if necessary. Take a breath and exhale slowly, putting the left heel down for the stretch. Hold the stretch for 15 seconds, breathing normally, and then slowly stand upright.

**Repetition.** The above is one full repetition of the quadriceps stretch.

**Advantages.** The first portion of this stretch pushes the knees outward, while keeping the palms together prevents overstretching.

**Disadvantages.** It is difficult to maintain balance when doing this stretch for the first time.

WARNINGS. Take care not to lose balance while doing this stretch. Make sure a support is available to grasp during the third and fourth steps to prevent a fall.

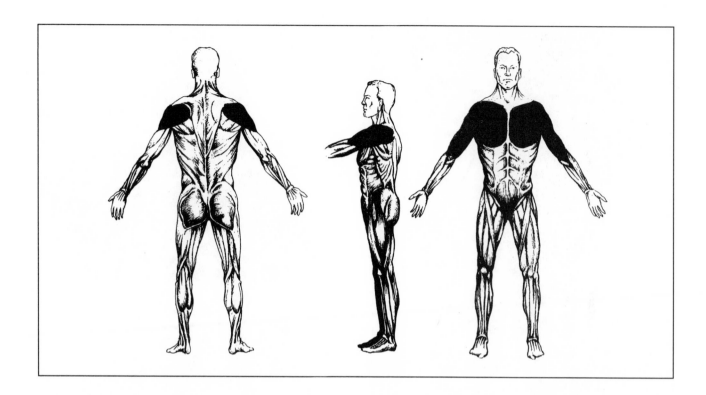

## SWIMMER (CHEST) STRETCH

**Muscle groups.** Chest, shoulders, and upper arms, especially the pectoralis major, deltoid, and biceps muscles.

   This stretch loosens and warms the muscles used in swimming with the arms. The angles of the arms during the stretch are specific for working the muscles for swimming.

### Technique

1. In an upright posture with the feet shoulder-width apart, swing both arms around behind the back. Interlace the fingers of the hands together with the palms facing each other. While leaning forward from the waist, raise the hands up behind the back, away from the body, into the up position while keeping the arms straight. Move the arms by rotating them at the shoulders to go into the stretch. The head remains straight on the neck, facing down, during the movement. Hold the arms in the up position for 15 seconds while breathing normally. Lower the arms and, while bending the knees slightly, return to the upright position.

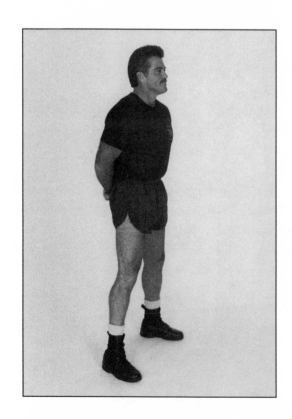

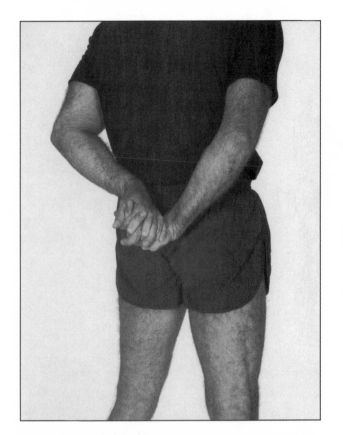

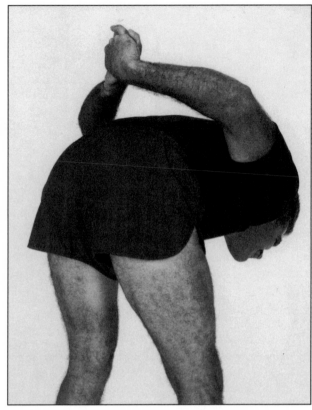

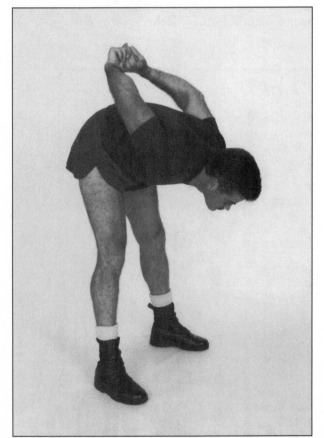

**Repetition.** The above completes one repetition of the swimmer stretch.

**Advantages.** This stretch works the chest, shoulders, and arm muscles that are also used in a number of weight lifting exercises (bench press, overhead press, etc.) as well as swimming.

**Disadvantages.** The movements of the arms behind the back can be difficult to do if the arm and shoulder muscles are tight or stiff. Take care when raising the arms to not cause pain in the chest or shoulders.

WARNINGS. Bend at the knees when straightening up from the stretch to minimize strain on the knees and lower back.

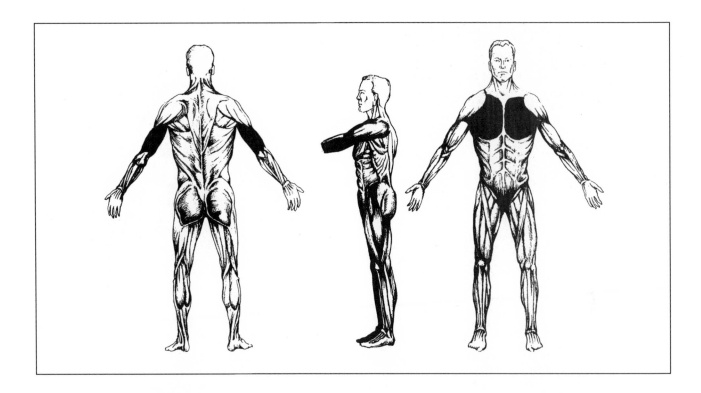

## TRICEPS STRETCH

**Muscle groups.** Underside of the upper arm and the chest, particularly the triceps and pectoralis major.

This is an important stretch for the upper body, which can greatly extend the movements of a group of muscles that are normally heavily worked during exercise.

### Technique

1. In an upright posture, raise the right arm and bend it at the elbow. Turn the arm so that the right hand can pass by the head while going over the right shoulder. Extend the upper right arm past the shoulder and down along the back of the head and spine. The right elbow should be pointing close to straight up from the shoulder. Reach around over the head with the left arm and grasp the right elbow with the left fingers. Pull the right arm back and down with the left hand for the stretch. Hold the stretch for 15 seconds while con-

tinuing to breathe normally. Slowly release the arms and move them back to the sides.

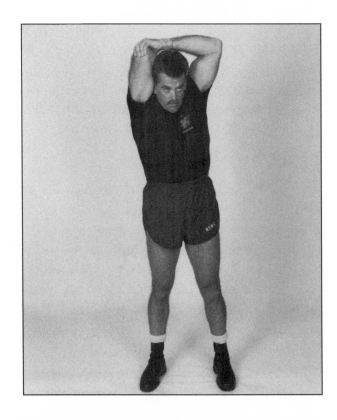

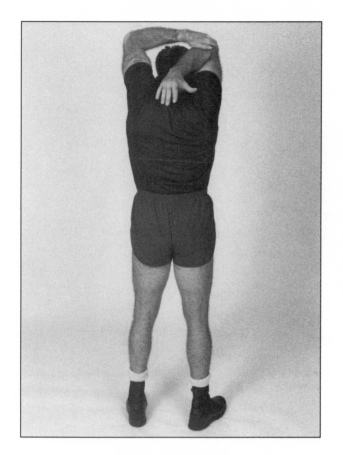

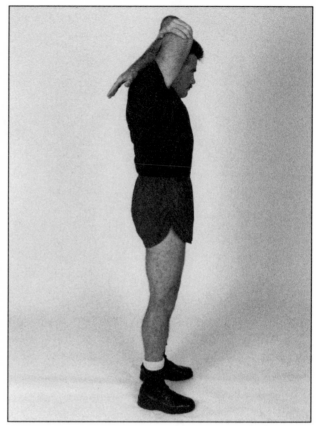

2. Reverse arms, putting the left arm up and bent behind the head. Reach over the head with the right arm and grasp the left elbow with the right fingers. Pull the left arm back and down into the stretch. Hold the stretch for 15 seconds while breathing normally and then release slowly.

*Note.* Additional muscles, including the latissimus dorsi and internal and external obliques, can be easily included in this stretch. As the arm is pressed back into the stretch, lean the torso to the opposite side of the arm being worked. When the right arm is up and pushed down behind the back, the lean would be to the left; when the left arm is pushed back, the lean would be to the right. Hold this stretch simultaneously with the arm stretch and for the same length of time.

**Repetition.** The above completes one full repetition of the triceps stretch.

**Advantages.** With a simple addition, this stretch can include most of the major muscle groups of the upper torso and side.

**Disadvantages.** This is a difficult stretch to perform if the muscles are already built up and stiff from previous exercise.

WARNINGS. Be sure the muscles are warmed up somewhat to minimize stiffness before doing this stretch. Do not push excessively on the elbow with the opposite hand to extend the stretch. Stop immediately at the point of pain anywhere in the shoulder, arm, or side.

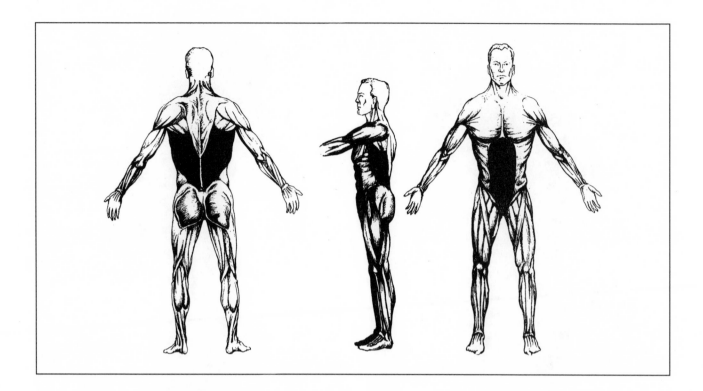

## TRUNK BENDING, FORE AND AFT

**Muscle groups.** Abdomen and lower back, including the rectus abdominus, latissimus dorsi, lumbodorsal fascia, and sacrospinalis.

This movement works the major muscles of the abdomen while particularly stretching and building up the lower-back muscles at a gradual rate.

### Technique

1. Stand upright with the feet shoulder-width apart. While bending the elbows outward, put the hands lightly on the hips, fingers forward, thumbs toward the back. Keep the eyes looking straight ahead. Taking a breath, exhale slowly and bend forward at the waist into the stretch. Hold the stretch for 15 seconds, keeping the head square on the shoulders and the eyes facing the floor. Keep the back straight during the stretch and bend slightly at the knees. Breathe normally during the stretch.

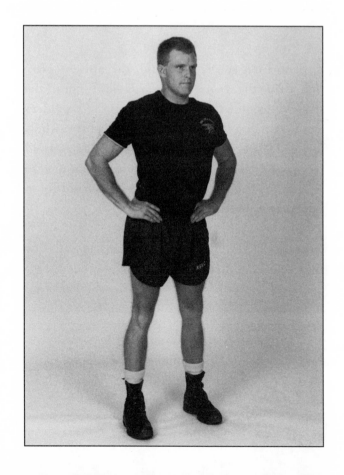

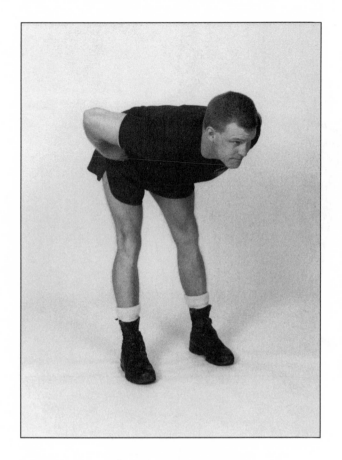 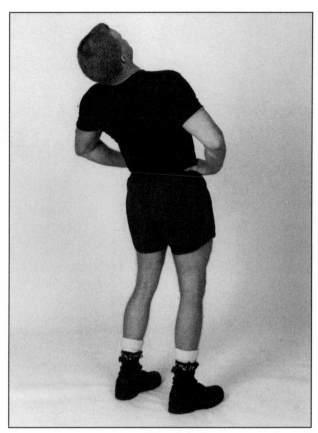

2. Straighten slowly back into the upright position. Tilt the body backward slowly into the stretch, keeping the head square to the shoulders and looking up toward the ceiling. Thrust the hips forward as needed to help maintain balance. Hold the stretch for 15 seconds while continuing to breathe normally. Relax and straighten slowly to the upright position.

**Repetition.** The above completes one repetition of the fore-and-aft trunk bend.

**Advantages.** This stretch will help build up the back muscles as well as maintain the flexibility of all the trunk muscles.

**Disadvantages.** Bending too far to the rear can compress disks in the back and otherwise injure it.

WARNINGS. To prevent hyperextending and possibly injuring the back when bending to the rear, keep the knees bent slightly. If there is any pain in the back at any point, stop the stretch immediately.

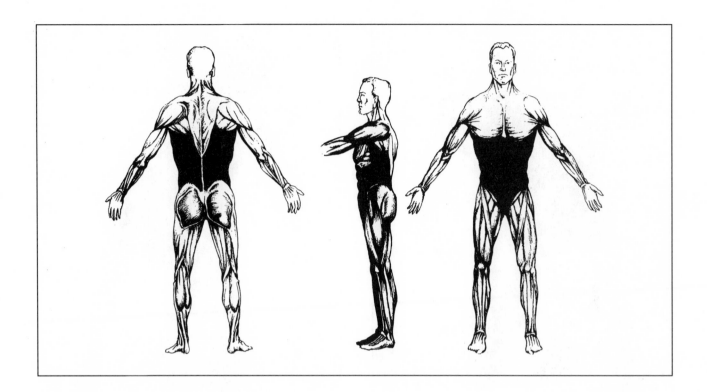

## TRUNK SIDE STRETCH

**Muscle groups.** Sides of the abdomen and the lower back, including the rectus abdominis, internal and external obliques, the latissimus dorsi, lumbodorsal fascia, and sacrospinalis.

This movement extends the muscles of the sides of the abdomen, increasing flexibility and the efficiency of breathing. At the same time, this stretch gradually builds up the strength of the lower back.

## Technique

1. Standing upright with the feet spread to about double shoulder-width apart, extend the left arm down the outside of the left leg, palm inward. As the trunk is leaned to the left, bending at the waist, slide the left arm down along the leg. The right arm is swung up as the lean begins and extended above the shoulder and bent over the head as the movement continues. The right forearm points with an open hand in the direction of the lean. The right side is stretched and the position held for 15 seconds. The head is facing forward during the movement and breathing remains normal. After the stretch, slowly return to the upright position.

2. The stretch is continued to the right. The right arm is extended down the outside of the right leg and the left arm swung up over the head during the movement. Hold the stretch for 15 seconds while breathing normally. Slowly straighten and return to the upright posture with a smooth motion.

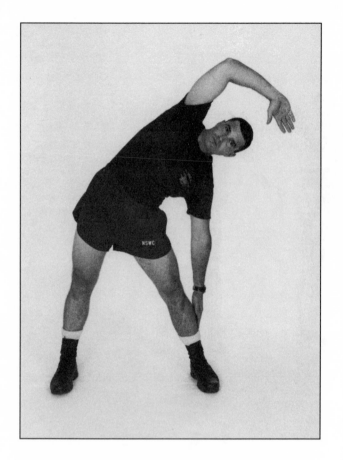
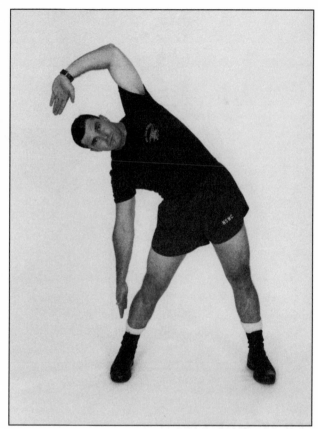

**Repetition.** The above completes one full repetition of the trunk side stretch.

**Advantages.** This movement gradually builds up the back muscles in strength and flexibility while extending the flexibility of the side obliques. The stretch also assists in pulling in the waistline.

**Disadvantages.** An excessive bend to the side can cause injury to the lower back by compression.

WARNINGS. Keep the back straight during the lean to minimize stress in the lower back.

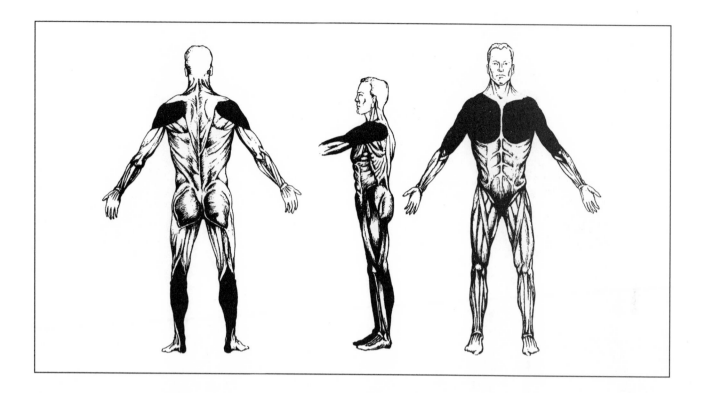

## UP, BACK, AND OVER

**Muscle groups.** Calves, shoulders, upper arms and chest, especially the gastrocnemius, soleus, and plantaris muscles, as well as the pectoralis majors, deltoids, and biceps.

This low-impact movement combines a dynamic action with a stretch increasing the overall effectiveness of the action.

## Technique

1. From the standing position with the feet shoulder-width apart and the arms hanging loosely to the sides, swing the arms forward and up and lift the heels of the feet several inches from the ground. The arms are stretched in the up position as they reach directly overhead. The upswing of the arms coincides with the lift of the legs up onto the balls of the feet. The up stretches in both the arms and feet are held for a short pause. (Up)

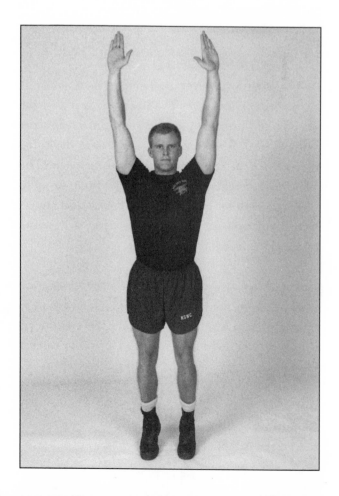

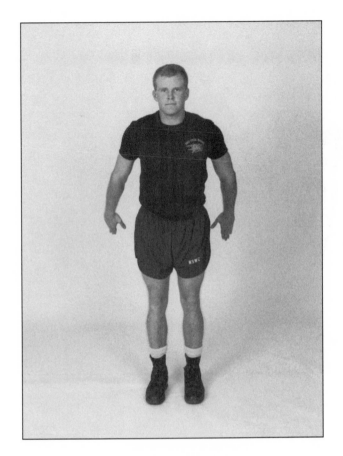
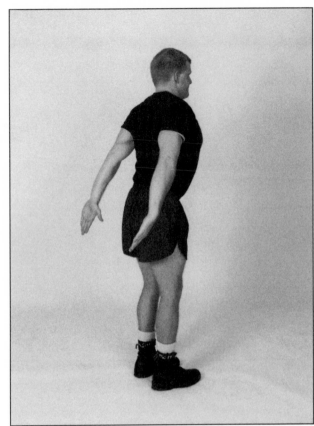

2. The heels of the feet are brought back down as the arms are lowered. The lowering swing of the arms is continued on past the body and to the rear. With the hands open and the arms straight, swing the arms to the rear and up behind the back. The arms are stretched up at the rear of their swing to their maximum reach. The back position stretch is held for a moment and then the arms are swung forward again. (Back)

3. On the forward movement of the arms, the swing is continued with the arms going over the head and into a full circle around the shoulders. The arms are held as straight as possible during the entire motion and the feet remain flat on the floor. (Over)

**Repetition.** The above completes one full repetition of the up, back, and over.

**Advantages.** This is a low-impact movement that includes most of the body in the action.

WARNINGS. Be certain there is enough overhead clearance for the arms to swing without striking anything.

## RUNNING STRETCHES

This group of stretches are especially useful to perform prior to and after a run. They are also used to loosen and warm the muscles for any actions that involve heavy use of the legs such as a lower-body workout or distance swim with fins.

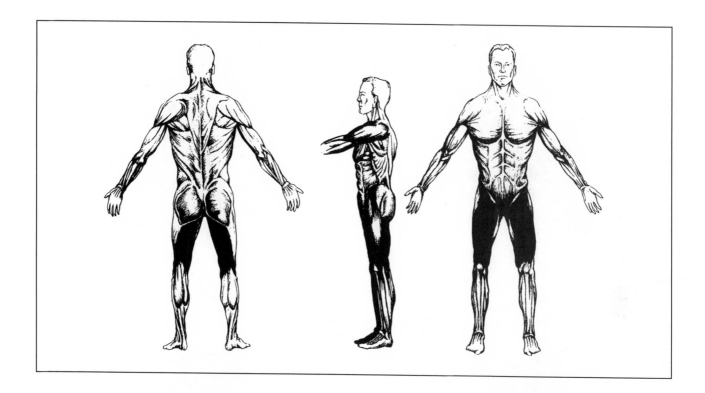

## HURDLER STRETCH

**Muscle groups.** Front and rear of the thighs, specifically the quadriceps femoris and hamstrings.

This is a difficult stretch for the legs but fully extends the thigh muscles with additional benefit to the lower back and calves.

### Technique

1. From the upright sitting position, extend the right leg with the toes of the foot pointed up. The left leg is bent at the knee and is turned to the side with the knee extending out and the foot flat against the inside of the right thigh. The left hand holds the toes of the left foot with the arm out over the bent left leg.

2. The right arm is extended forward, along the top of the right leg as the trunk is bent forward from the waist. With the head held straight, take a breath and exhale slowly while leaning the body

into the stretch. During the movement, grasp the right toes with the right hand and pull the top of the foot back toward the body to stretch the calf. The left elbow presses gently down on the left leg during the stretch. Hold the stretch for 15 seconds while breathing normally. Relax and return to the upright sitting position.

3. Switch the position of the legs, extending the left leg out and bringing the right leg back into the bent position. The right foot is now flat against the inside of the left thigh. The right hand holds the toes of the right foot with the arm out over the bent leg.

4. Extend the left arm forward above the leg as the trunk is bent forward from the waist. With the head held straight, take a breath and exhale slowly while leaning the body into the stretch. During the movement, grasp the left toes with the left hand and pull the top of the foot back toward

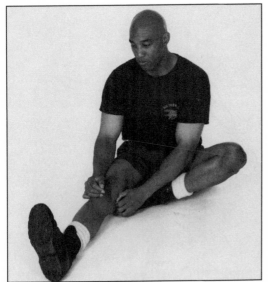

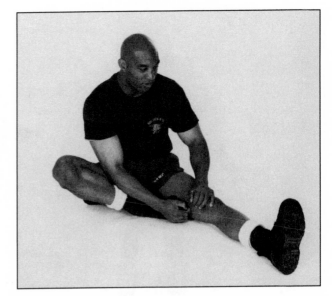

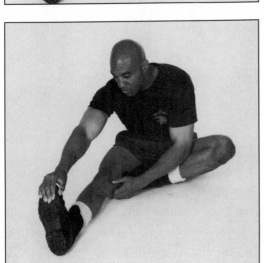

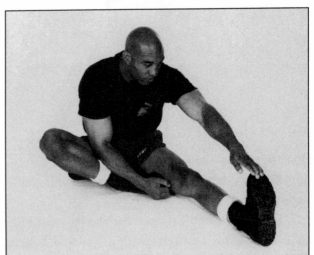

the body to stretch the calf. The right elbow presses gently down on the right leg during the stretch. Hold the stretch for 15 seconds while breathing normally. Relax and return to the upright sitting position.

**Repetition.** The above completes one full repetition of the hurdler stretch.

**Advantages.** This stretch extends the upper leg muscles to their maximum extent.

**Disadvantages.** This is a difficult stretch to do. Stress can be high on the bent leg when it is pressed down by the arm. It is difficult to inhale while in the forward lean portion of this movement.

WARNINGS. Do not press down hard or bounce the bent leg during this movement to increase the stretch.

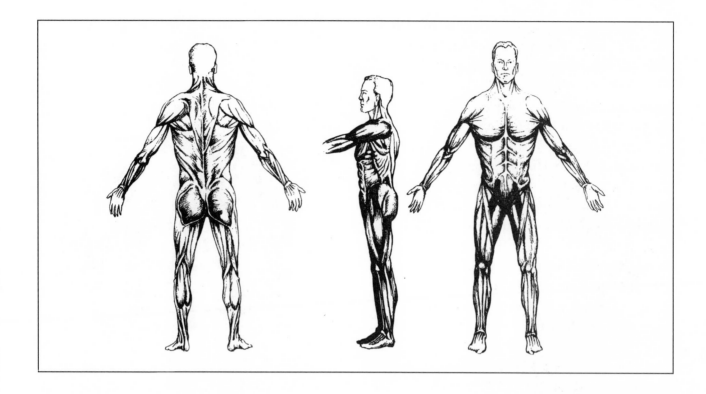

## GROIN (BUTTERFLY) STRETCH

**Muscle groups.** Groin and inside thigh, especially the psoas major; iliacus; gracilis; and the adductor longus, brevis, and magus muscles.

This is an advanced movement for the groin and is one of the most effective stretches for that area of the body.

### Technique

1. While in the upright sitting position, bring the knees up in front of the chest, keeping the feet together and flat on the floor. Spread the knees apart and place the soles of the feet together. With the arms going between the knees, grasp the feet with both hands and draw the heels in to the groin area.

Take a breath and exhale slowly, leaning forward into the hands while spreading the knees apart. The arms may also be used to spread the knees lightly or the knees may be gently wiggled up and

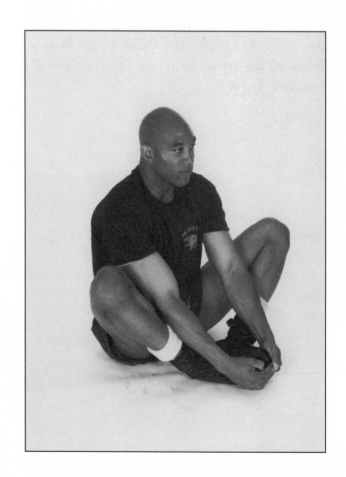

down without bouncing them. Try to bend from the waist while pulling up on the feet. Breathe normally and hold the stretch for 15 seconds.

**Repetition.** The above completes one repetition of the butterfly groin stretch.

**Advantages.** A very effective stretch for the groin area. The movement can be continued over time until the knees can be placed flat on the floor and the heels drawn fully in to the groin.

**Disadvantages.** This is a very difficult stretch to complete until some flexibility is built up in the groin and thighs. It is easy to overstretch and cause injury with this movement.

WARNINGS. Do not try to bring the feet in too closely to the groin as this can overstress the knees. Do not force the knees down with the arms but only press gently. If wiggling the knees up and down, do the motion gently and do not bounce. Bouncing can easily cause an injury, especially with this stretch.

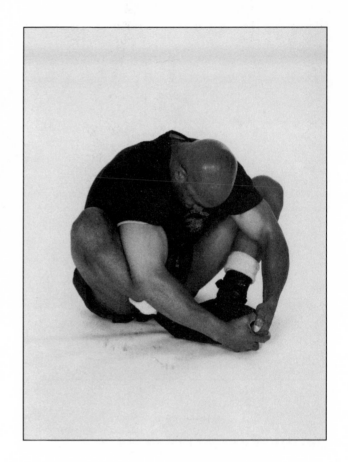

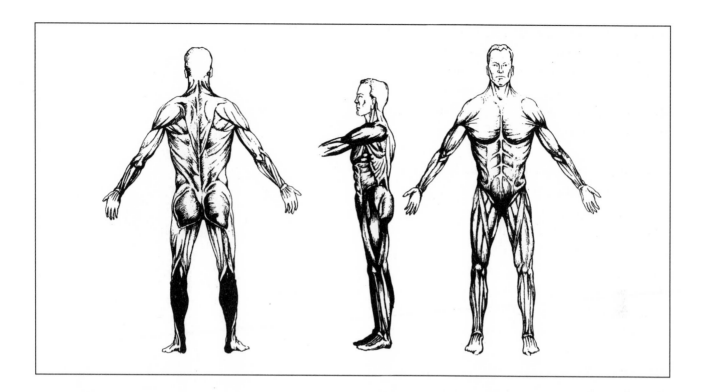

## CALF/ACHILLES STRETCH

**Muscle groups.** Back of the lower leg, particularly the gastrocnemius, soleus, and plantaris muscles as well as the Achilles tendon.

This stretch is one of the standards when preparing for a run or swim. It both strengthens and loosens the lower leg and foot.

### Technique

1. Stand upright facing a wall or other support. Lean forward, bracing the arms with the hands flat on the support. Bring the left leg forward, bending it at the knee, and rest the foot on the ground. Extend the right leg fully to the rear, to the maximum point where the sole of the foot is still flat on the floor. Bend the arms and left leg slowly, bringing the hips forward while still keeping the right foot flat on the floor. The stretch should be felt in the calf and on the back of the ankle on the rear leg. Hold a firm stretch for 15 seconds while breathing normally and then relax.

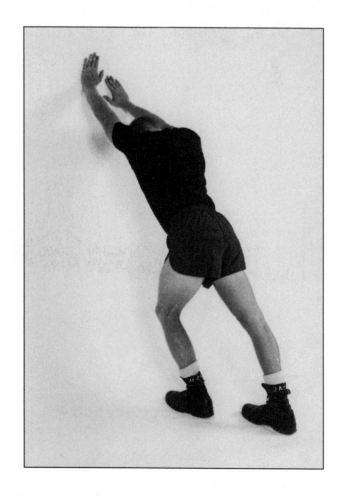

2. With the arms remaining in position, switch legs with the right leg now being bent at the knee and forward and the left leg extending to the rear. With the left leg straight to the rear and the foot flat on the floor, slowly lean forward into the stretch. Hold the stretch for 15 seconds and relax.

**Repetition.** The above is one full repetition of the calf/Achilles tendon stretch.

**Advantages.** This movement helps add both flexibility and energy to the legs.

**Disadvantages.** This stretch should only be done against a solid support. Overstretching is easy with this movement so extra care should be taken.

WARNINGS. Do not overstretch. The Achilles tendon only needs a slight stretch for improvement. An overstretch can quickly create a very painful situation that can be a long time healing.

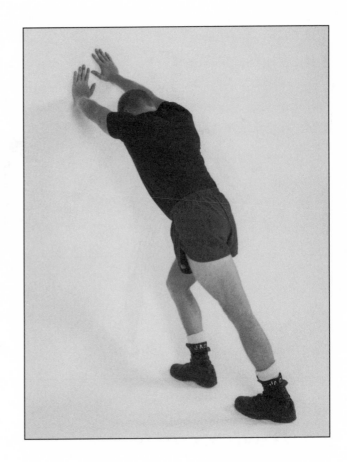

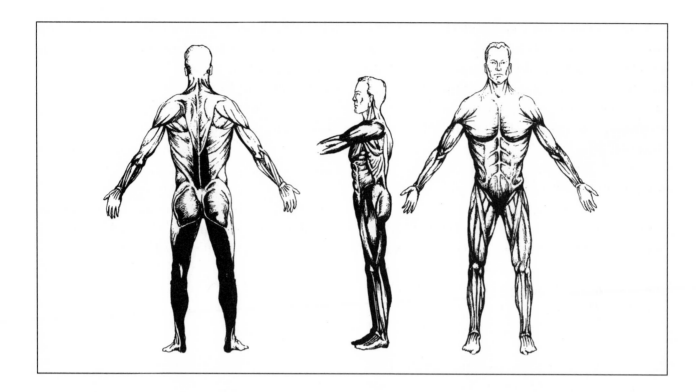

## SITTING CALF/HAMSTRING STRETCH

**Muscle groups.** Rear of the thigh and the back of the lower leg, particularly the hamstrings and the gastrocnemius, soleus, and plantaris muscles as well as the Achilles tendon, lumbodorsal fascia, and sacrospinalis muscles.

This sitting stretch pulls the muscles at the rear of the leg without the strain of some of the standing stretches. There is also some benefit to the lower back and outer abdominal muscles. This stretch is the standard used to improve performance on the military sit-reach test.

### Technique

1. In the sitting position, extend the legs straight out and hold them together. The feet are held with the toes pointed up. Reach out and grasp the toes of the feet while keeping the legs straight and the backs of the knees flat on the ground. If the toes cannot be reached with the hands, use a towel or other object looped around the toes to extend the

reach of the arms. The towel may be used to develop the flexibility needed to complete the stretch without aid.

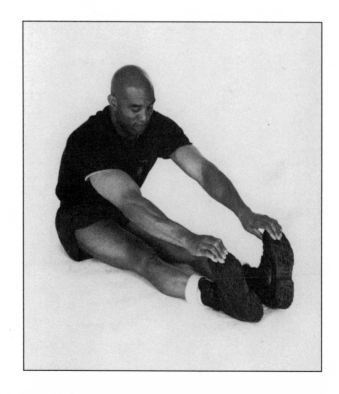

2. Take a deep breath and pull back with the hands on the slow exhale. Keep the back as straight as possible and bend from the hips. Pull the toes back for the stretch, keeping the legs straight and the knees against the ground. Hold the stretch for 15 seconds while breathing normally and relax.

**Repetition.** The above is one repetition of the sitting calf/hamstring stretch.

**Advantages.** This movement can be used to build up to more strenuous stretches. The stretch is felt first in the back of the knees and throughout the back of the lower leg. Keeping the toes pointed up increases the stretch for the calf muscles. Using an extension, such as a towel, allows the full stretch to be easily built up to.

**Disadvantages.** Pulling back too hard can overstretch the Achilles tendon and the muscles of the calves.

WARNINGS. Do not overstretch the Achilles tendon by pulling back excessively on the toes. The heels only have to be slightly raised off the ground for the stretch.

# CALISTHENICS

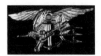

After Hell Week our real technical training began.
The difficulties of Hell Week help UDTR and BUD/S to weed out
those individuals who don't have the intestinal fortitude
to make it to the Teams before the Navy spends
a great deal of money on their training.
—SEAL, Class 27

THOUGH WEIGHT TRAINING, both with free weights and machines, is a beneficial course of exercise, the best workouts to use in preparing for BUD/S involve calisthenics that center on moving the body's own weight. These exercises are considered isotonic training. An isotonic contraction is one where the muscle contracts and shortens while movement is taking place. Whenever an individual does a calisthenic exercise or moves a weight, an isotonic contraction takes place.

With calisthenics, the exercises often involve the entire body, even where only a portion of the body is actually undergoing movement. The actions of maintaining balance and holding the rest of the body still involves the work of a great many muscles. It is this general action that adds greatly to the overall effectiveness of a series of calisthenic exercises.

## UPPER BODY EXERCISES

❏

STANDARD PUSH-UP

STANDARD PULL-UP

REVERSE GRIP PULL-UP
(CHIN-UPS)

WIDE GRIP PULL-UP

SIDE-TO-SIDE PULL-UP
(COMMANDO PULL-UPS)

HANGING KNEE-UPS, RIGHT/LEFT
SIDE

HANGING KNEE-UPS, STRAIGHT

DIPS

NECK ROTATIONS

❏

## LEG EXERCISES

❏

CALF RAISES

LUNGES

STAR JUMPERS

HALF-DEEP KNEE BENDS (TOUCH
YOUR BOOTS)

STOMACH FLUTTER KICKS

❏

## GENERAL

❏

EIGHT-COUNT BODY BUILDERS

❏

## ABDOMINAL EXERCISES

❏

STANDARD SIT-UP

HALF SIT-UPS

CROSS-LEG SIT-UPS, RIGHT/LEFT
(CROSSOVERS)

EXTENDED LEG CRUNCHES

BENT LEG CRUNCHES

RAISED BENT LEG CRUNCHES

TRUNK ROTATIONS

HIP THRUST (PELVIC TILT)

WAVE-OFFS

LEG LEVERS

KNEE-UPS

❏

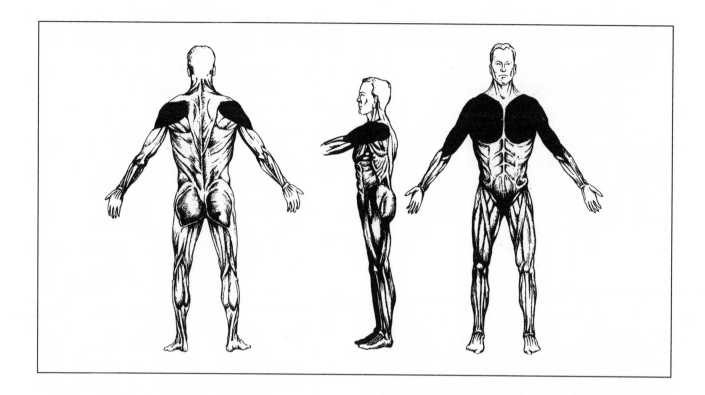

## STANDARD PUSH-UP

**Muscle groups.** Upper body including the shoulders, arms, chest, and back, especially the pectoralis major, deltoid, and biceps muscles.

For both practical and some traditional reasons, the standard push-up is the most common calisthenic exercise performed in the U.S. military. This exercise develops upper-body strength in the chest, shoulders, and arms with the muscles lifting about 70 percent of the individual's body weight. Modified forms of the push-up are also able to concentrate development of some specific muscle groups.

## Technique

1. Begin in the "front leaning rest" position. Feet are held together, supported by the toes on the ground. The legs are held straight and even with the back. The hands are placed palms down, fingers forward, with the spacing of the hands being slightly greater than shoulder-width (sufficient to clear the sides of the chest). The head is held up with the eyes looking forward.

2. Lower your body to the floor by bending the elbows and rotating the shoulders. Keep the legs and back straight during all phases of the exercise. Stop lowering your body when your chest lightly touches the floor. (Count 1)

3. Push the upper body back up to the starting position with a smooth motion, keeping the legs and back straight. (Count 2)

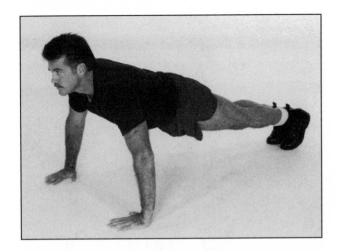

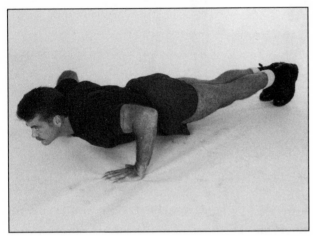

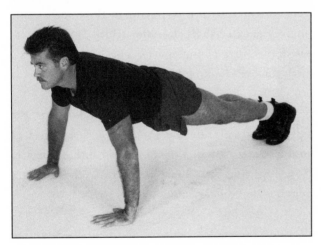

**Advantages.** The push-up can be conducted under almost any circumstances where there is a firm surface to lie on. This includes doing the exercise in the surf where the head clears the water only in the up position. Push-ups are excellent for the buildup of general upper-body strength with some additional aerobic cardiovascular benefits when conducted in larger repetitions done rapidly.

**Disadvantages.** Increases in resistance for the push-up require additional weight be added onto the back of the individual. This is very hard to do while exercising alone. A sandbag-filled backpack is one way of adding additional weight for the exercise. A raised platform such as a step, block, or chair can be used to elevate the feet for an even more difficult exercise. Raising the feet increases the percentage of the body weight being lifted to 78 to 80 percent of the individual's weight.

Doing a push-up with the legs highly elevated, such as a "handstand" or inverted push-up done with the legs supported against a wall, increases the intensity of the exercise to its maximum while concentrating the force needed from the arms and shoulders. An inverted push-up forces the muscles of the upper body to lift very close to 100 percent of the individual's weight.

WARNINGS. Do not bend the back or raise the buttocks during the exercise. Also do not hang the waist down while supporting the upper body with the arms. Few injuries can result from the execution of a standard push-up done with the toes resting on the ground. Raising the feet on a taller rest increases the chances of muscle strain or slipping and striking the ground.

**Repetition.** The above completes a single repetition of a two-count push-up. A four-count push-up, commonly used during PT sessions, includes a repeat of steps 2 and 3 to complete a single repetition.

## PULL-UPS

All pull-ups and their variations require some kind of suspended bar to complete correctly. Commercial chin-up bars that can be mounted in a doorway are on the market. The bars available include those solidly screwed into the doorframe and removable models that are held by brackets. The doorway-mounted bar has one major drawback in that it is usually too low to allow a deadhang from the bar with the legs and arms straight with the feet clear of the floor.

An individual can clear enough distance on a doorway-mounted bar to properly perform the exercises by lifting his legs clear of the floor. Lift the legs by bending at the knee rather than by trying to lift forward from the hip. By crossing the ankles, you can lock the legs together, which aids in maintaining the bent-leg position.

Most school gymnasiums, playgrounds, and health clubs have standing chin-up bars available or other structures suitable for use. Military requirements for a chin-up bar call for two or more 6- by 6-inch square wooden posts, mounted in the ground and extending up to a height of 8 feet 6 inches. The supports must remain rigidly upright and need to be firmly set into the ground, spaced 5 feet apart.

The horizontal bar on a military setup is made from a length of smooth steel pipe, usually galvanized water pipe, with a $1\frac{1}{2}$-inch outside diameter. The pipe is passed through holes drilled in the upright supports, 6 inches down from the top of each post. The pipe is secured so that it cannot turn during use. In some cases the pipe is covered with heavy cloth tape for additional grip and to protect the hands. Step-up blocks are attached to the inside of each support post with the top of the blocks being 18 inches above the ground.

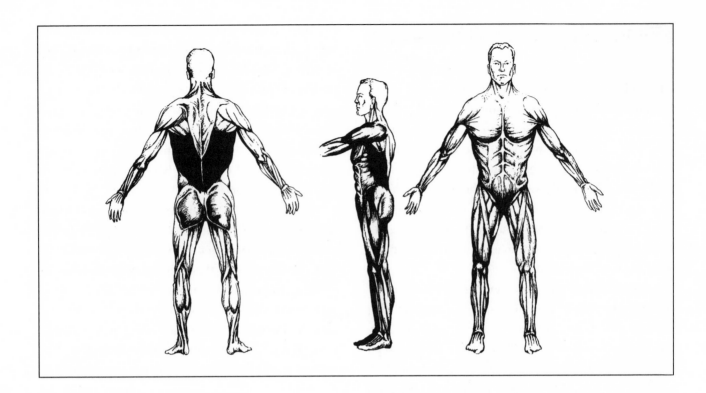

## STANDARD PULL-UP

**Muscle groups.** Arms, hands, chest, and back, especially the latissimus dorsi along the mid-back and sides.

This exercise is one of the most effective at building up the shoulders, arms, and upper back. Just changing the way the bar is held and the spacing of the hands increases or decreases the difficulty of the exercise and forces concentration of effort on specific muscle groups. It is also one of the hardest exercises to perform properly with repetition.

One of the most common reasons for failing to pass the initial BUD/S screening test is the inability to complete 6 perfect dead-hang pull-ups. It takes a minimum of 6 completed pull-ups to qualify for BUD/S training. It is highly recommended that a prospective student be able to complete 15 correct pull-ups before entering training.

**Technique**

1. Stand at the pull-up bar and grasp the bar with a pronated grip (palms facing away from your face). The hands should be spaced slightly greater than shoulder-width apart. Hang the body down from the bar in a dead-hang position, with the elbows straight and the full weight of the body pulling on the hands. If the legs do not clear the ground in the dead-hang starting position, raise the feet by bending the lower legs back at the knees. Crossing the ankles can add to stability when in the bent-leg position.

2. Raise the body up in a single, smooth motion, pulling the bar down toward your chest, until your chin is above the bar. Do not bicycle (lift the feet alternately) or kick the legs while lifting the body. Exhale on the up motion. (Count 1)

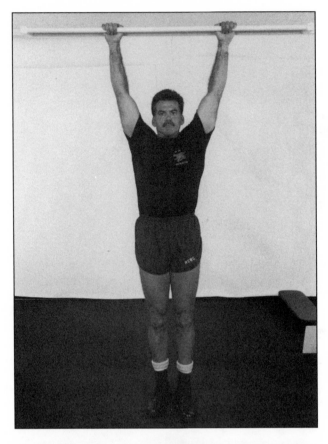

3. While maintaining control, slowly and smoothly lower the body down from the bar until the arms are back in their fully-extended position (dead hang). (Count 2)

**Repetition.** The above completes a single repetition of a two-count pull-up.

**Advantages.** This basic exercise is a tremendous general aid in building up the muscles of the upper body including those of the back. Even if not completed, attempting the exercise and raising the body partway to the bar has some benefit in strength development.

**Disadvantages.** This is a very difficult exercise to complete. A firmly supported pull-up bar is a necessity or the exercise cannot be completed properly.

WARNINGS. It is very easy to overexert yourself when performing this exercise for the first time. Pace your development carefully and use a lower number of repetitions, correctly completed, to gradually build yourself up.

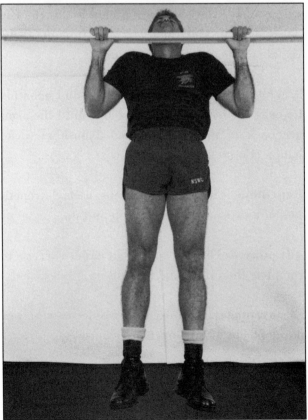

TIP. As an aid to initial pull-up workouts, use a chair or other support for the legs. Use any solid means of support that is as high as your knees when hanging from the bar in the starting position. Putting the support a short distance behind you allows you to place your feet on the support when your legs are bent. That will enable you to use some of the strength in your legs to assist in lifting your body weight when beginning a course of exercise involving the pull-up. Remember to lift the feet free of the support and lower them back to the ground before letting go of the bar.

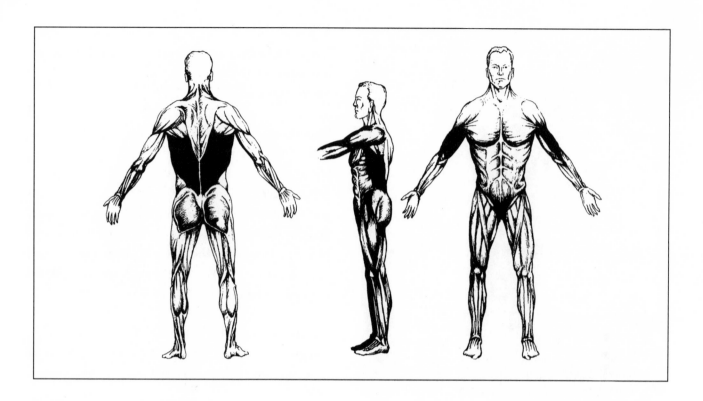

## REVERSE GRIP PULL-UP (CHIN-UP)

**Muscle groups.** Arms, hands, chest, and back, especially the latissimus dorsi muscle along the mid-back and sides and the biceps on the upper arm.

This is a slightly easier exercise to properly complete than the standard pull-up. Reversing the grip gives a mechanical advantage to the biceps muscle allowing it to more easily lift the body's weight.

### Technique

1. Stand at the pull-up bar and grasp the bar with a supinated grip (palms facing in, toward your face). The hands should be spaced out above the shoulder or slightly greater than shoulder-width apart. Hang the body down from the bar in a dead-hang position, with the elbows straight and the full weight of the body pulling on the hands.

2. Raise the body up in a single, smooth motion, pulling the bar down toward your chest, until your chin is above the bar. Do not bicycle (lift the feet alternately) or kick the legs while lifting the body. Exhale on the up motion. (Count 1)

3. While maintaining control, slowly and smoothly lower the body down from the bar until the arms are back in their fully-extended position (dead hang). (Count 2)

**Repetition.** The above completes a single repetition of a two-count reverse grip pull-up.

**Advantages.** This is a somewhat easier exercise to complete than the standard pull-up.

**Disadvantages.** The exercise results in a slower development of the upper-body muscles.

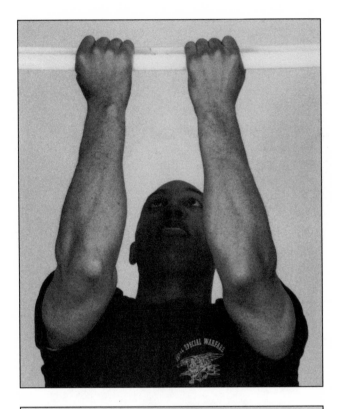

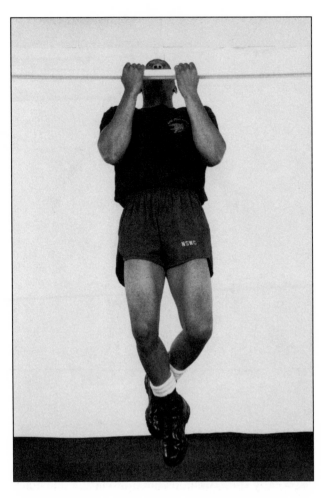

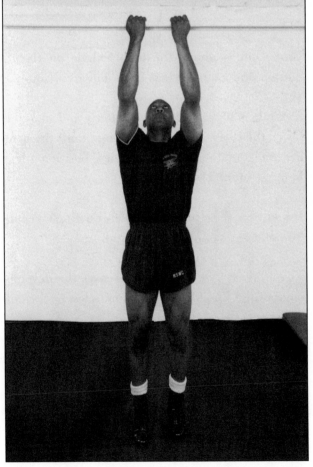

**Uses.** Use the reverse grip pull-up to aid in the development of the biceps as part of a regular workout routine. The exercise is especially useful in developing the strength needed to complete the regular pull-up. Use the reverse grip pull-up until 15 repetitions can be completed properly. Then begin using a lower number of standard pull-ups in your exercise routine.

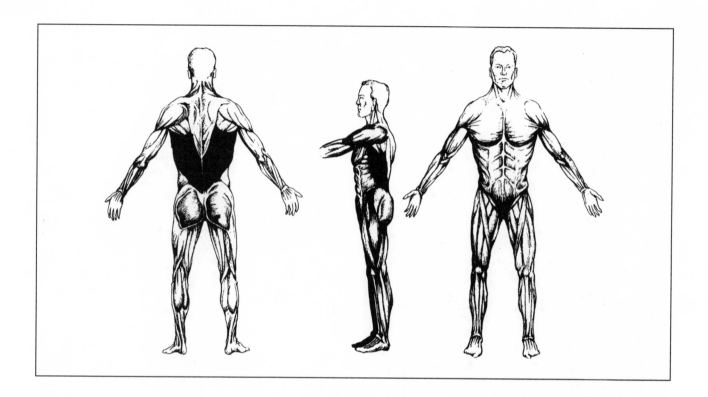

## WIDE GRIP PULL-UP

**Muscle groups.** Arms, hands, chest, and back, especially the latissimus dorsi along the mid-back and sides.

This exercise places most of the muscle groups of the shoulders and arms at a mechanical disadvantage. This disadvantage increases the work done by the muscles in moving the body's weight upward.

### Technique

1. Stand at the pull-up bar and grasp the bar with a pronated grip. The hands should be spaced almost double shoulder-width apart. Hang the body down from the bar in a dead-hang position, with the elbows straight, the arms in a V position, and the full weight of the body pulling on the hands.

2. Raise the body up in a single, smooth motion, pulling the bar down toward your chest, until your chin is above the bar. Exhale on the up motion and keep the legs from moving. (Count 1)

3. While maintaining control, slowly and smoothly lower the body down from the bar until the arms are back in their fully extended position (dead hang). (Count 2)

**Repetition.** The above completes a single repetition of a two-count wide grip pull-up.

**Advantages.** This exercise increases the development of the shoulder and arm muscles.

**Disadvantages.** It is a very hard exercise to complete and can quickly strain the muscles of the upper back, shoulders, and arms.

WARNINGS. Watch for excessive muscle strain.

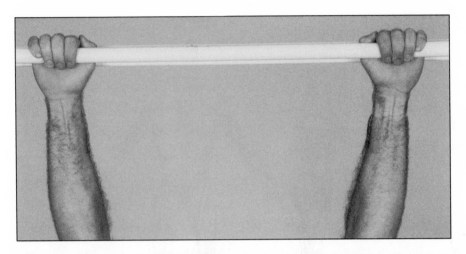

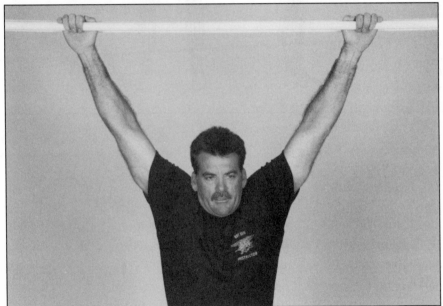

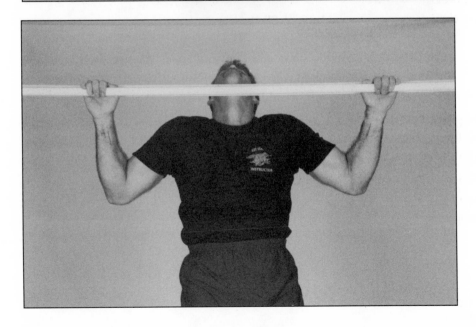

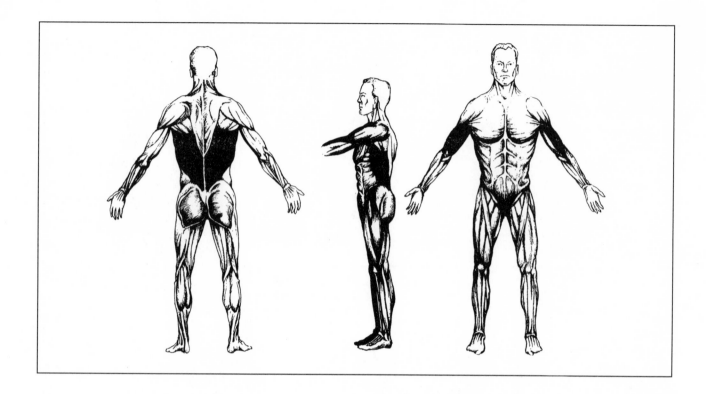

## SIDE-TO-SIDE PULL-UP (COMMANDO PULL-UP)

**Muscle groups.** Arms, hands, chest, and back, especially the latissimus dorsi muscle along the mid-back and sides and the biceps on the upper arm.

This is a harder exercise to complete than the reverse grip pull-up (chin-up) but concentrates the work done by the biceps muscles.

### Technique

1. Stand at the side of the bar, facing parallel with it. Grasp the bar with the hands close together so that one hand is palm-out to the left and one hand is palm-in to the right. The thumb of one hand should be just touching the pinkie of the other hand. Hang the body down from the bar with the arms straight in a dead-hang position.

2. Smoothly raise the body up to the left of the bar until the right shoulder touches the bar itself. (Count 1)

3. Lower the body slowly to the dead-hang position. (Count 2)

4. Raise the body up in a smooth motion to the right side of the bar. Stop lifting the body when the left shoulder touches the bar. (Count 3)

5. Slowly lower the body back down to the dead-hang starting position. (Count 4)

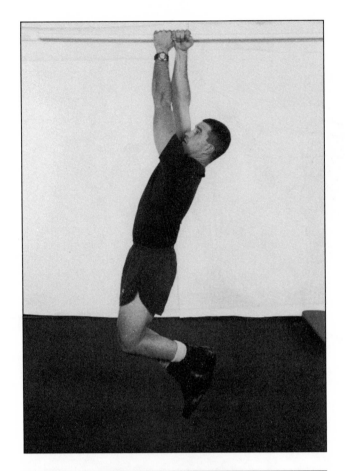

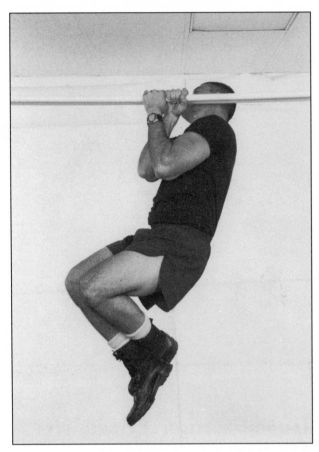

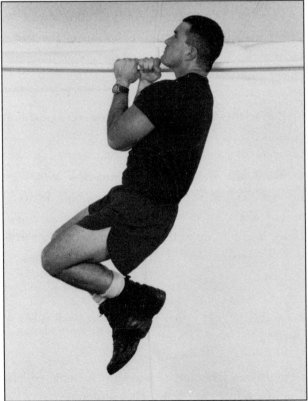

**Repetition.** Lifting the body up and touching first one shoulder, then lowering the body and raising it again and touching the opposite shoulder, makes one repetition of the four-count exercise.

**Advantages.** This exercise concentrates effort on first one and then the other biceps muscle. It increases the work put out by the biceps muscles while maintaining a difficult exercise.

**Disadvantages.** The exercise requires a long pull-up bar with a 5-foot spacing between supports.

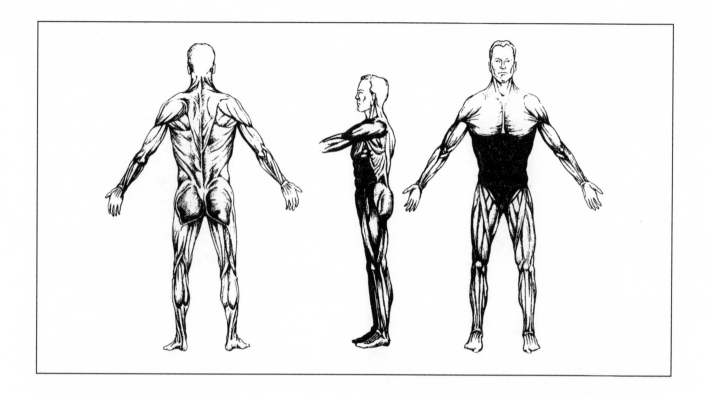

## HANGING KNEE-UPS, RIGHT/LEFT SIDE

**Muscle groups.** Upper and lower abdominals and obliques, specifically the rectus abdominis, transversalis abdominis, and internal and external obliques.

This exercise, which can be done on the same basic bar assembly as the pull-up, has a lighter, though noticeable, impact on the lower back while strongly working all of the abdominal muscles.

### Technique

1. Hang from the pull-up bar with the feet free of the floor and the hands in a comfortable position, spaced slightly greater than shoulder-width apart. If the feet do not clear the floor when hanging from the bar, the knees can be bent with the legs to the rear.

2. Bend the legs while bringing the knees up toward the right shoulder. Roll the hips up and forward as the knees bend past the 90-degree angle. Hold the knees up at the top of the movement with a full contraction of the abdominal muscles. (Count 1)

3. Lower the legs slowly to the starting position. (Count 2)

4. Bend the legs while bringing the knees up toward the left shoulder. Roll the hips forward and up as the knees bend past the 90-degree angle. Hold the knees up at the top of the movement with a full contraction of the abdominal muscles. (Count 3)

5. Lower the legs slowly to the floor, back into the starting position. (Count 4)

**Repetition.** The above completes a single repetition of a four-count right/left knee-up.

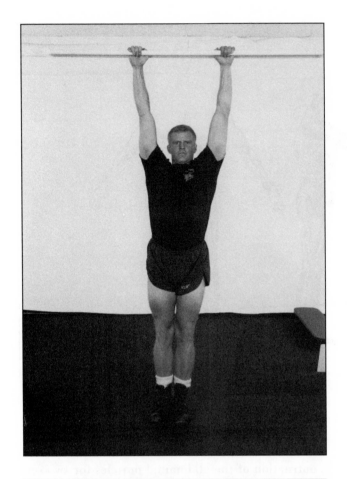

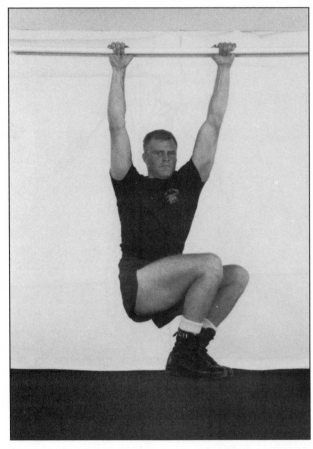

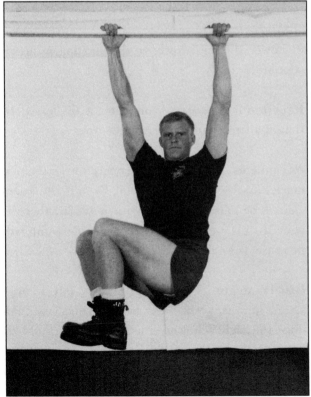

**Advantages.** This exercise strongly works the obliques as well as the other muscles of the abdomen. Even if the knees cannot be raised to a fully-up position, there is benefit to the exercise. The range of motion will increase as work is continued.

**Disadvantages.** This exercise does put a mild strain on the lower-back muscles and is a fairly difficult movement to complete. The body must be held still throughout the exercise without any forward swinging to build momentum. A firmly supported pull-up bar is necessary to complete this exercise.

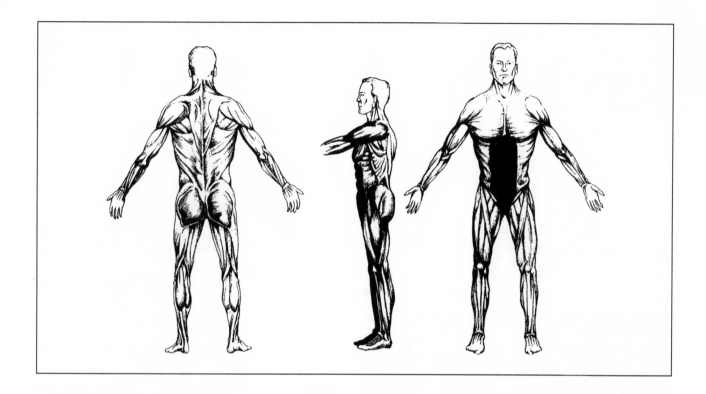

## HANGING KNEE-UPS, STRAIGHT

**Muscle groups.** Upper and lower abdominals with some effect on the obliques, specifically the rectus abdominis, and transversalis abdominis muscles.

Using the same bar assembly as the pull-up, this exercise has a higher impact on the lower back than the right/left hanging knee-up and strongly works the abdominal muscles.

### Technique

1. Hang from the pull-up bar with the feet free of the floor and the hands in a comfortable position, spaced slightly greater than shoulder-width apart. If the feet do not clear the floor when hanging from the bar, the knees can be bent with the legs to the rear.

2. Bend the legs while bringing the knees straight up toward the chest. Roll the hips up and forward as the knees bend past the 90-degree angle. Hold the knees up at the top of the movement with a full

contraction of the abdominal muscles for two seconds. (Count 1)

3. Lower the legs slowly to the starting position. (Count 2)

**Repetition.** The above completes a single repetition of a two-count straight knee-up.

**Advantages.** This exercise strongly works the primary muscles of the abdomen. Even if the knees cannot be raised to a fully-up position, there is benefit to the exercise. The range of motion will increase as work is continued.

**Disadvantages.** This exercise does put a mild strain on the lower-back muscles but less than does the right/left knee-ups. The body must be held still through the exercise without any forward swinging to build momentum. A firmly supported pull-up bar is necessary to complete this exercise.

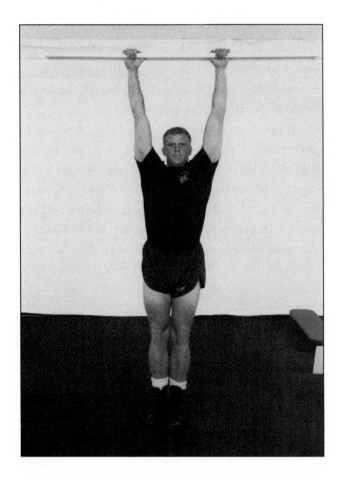

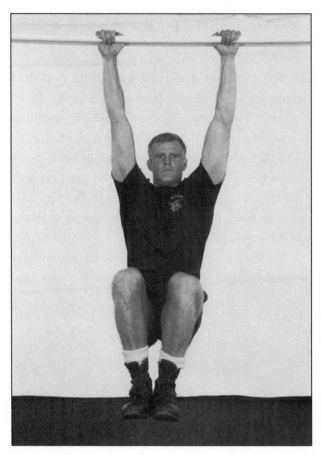

WARNINGS. A more difficult version of this exercise is the straight leg/hanging leg raise. The straight leg version is done with the legs held straight throughout the movement of the exercise and is otherwise the same as that of the straight knee-up.

The straight leg/hanging leg raise works the abdominal muscles to a greater extent than the hanging knee-up but puts the lower back at a much higher risk of injury.

## DIPS

All dip exercises and their variations require a secure set of parallel supports to properly do the exercise. The best equipment on which to do dips is a set of parallel bars, 1½ inches in diameter, set 24 to 28 inches apart (slightly greater than shoulder-width) and running 4 feet above the ground. Children's playground horizontal ladders can often be used to perform dips on as can a school gymnasium's parallel bars.

A satisfactory set of bars can be made up of several lengths of 1½-inch galvanized water pipe secured to uprights. The uprights can themselves be made up of the same or larger diameter water pipe with flanges on the bottom to secure them to a foundation and 90-degree elbows at the top to hold the horizontal pipe sections.

If no other apparatus is available, dips can be performed with two sturdy chairs. Make certain that the chairs are in good condition and easily capable of supporting your weight and remaining stable on the floor. Place the chairs slightly greater than shoulder-width apart, backs facing in the same direction, and perform the dips facing in the direction of the front of the chairs with your hands on top of the side of the chair's seat.

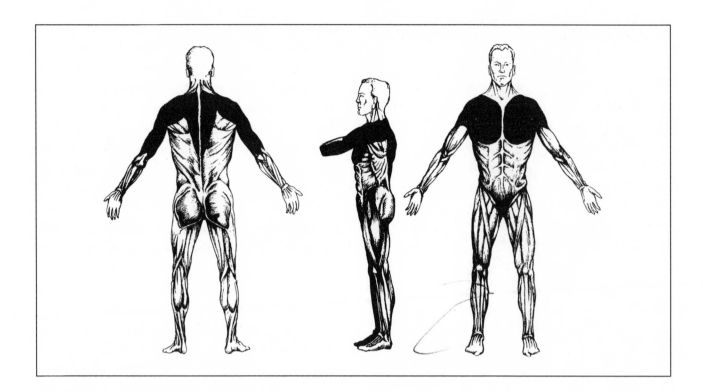

## DIPS

**Muscle groups.** Upper chest, shoulders, and arms concentrating on the pectoralis major, trapezius, deltoid, and triceps muscles.

Dips are among the most effective exercises for developing upper-body strength and are correspondingly hard to complete. Primary development is in the pectoral muscles of the chest but all of the upper body is involved in doing the exercise.

### Technique

1. Grasp two solid supports with your hands and lift the body up until the elbows are straight. The legs should not touch the ground at any time during the exercise. If the supports are too low to keep the legs clear of the ground, bend the lower legs backward at the knee. Crossing the ankles will help lock the legs together during the exercise.

2. Slowly lower the body by bending the arms until the elbows are turned to a 90-degree angle. Keep the legs from touching the ground and the body still and balanced. (Count 1)

3. Raise the body back up to the starting position in a single, smooth movement. (Count 2)

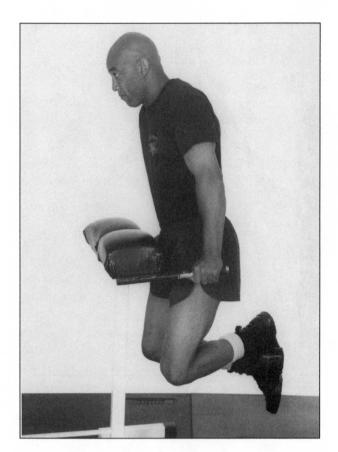

**Repetition.** The above completes a single repetition of a two-count dip.

**Advantages.** This is a very efficient exercise for building up the upper body with emphasis on the pectoral muscles. Even if a full dip movement cannot be completed, a partial movement is still beneficial to the muscles and will aid in building up the upper body.

**Disadvantages.** This exercise must be done with secure and steady supports for the hands.

WARNINGS. Supports used for dips must be able to easily support the full weight of the exerciser. They must also be stable and not move during the full range of motions conducted. Makeshift supports such as light chairs and other objects can suddenly fail during the exercise possibly causing serious injury.

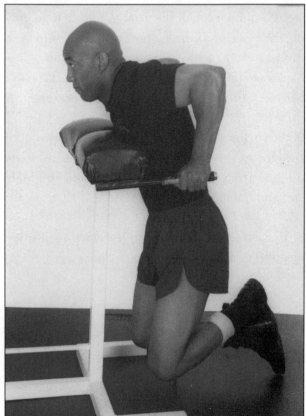

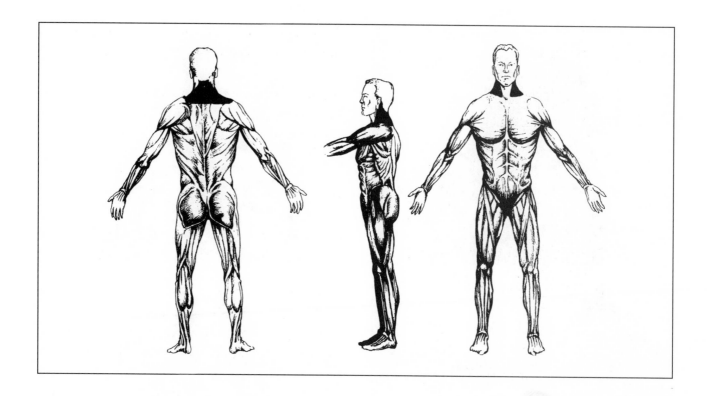

## NECK ROTATIONS

**Muscle groups.** Neck and upper shoulders, especially the upper trapezius, levator scapulae, and sternomastoid muscles.

This exercise works the muscles of the neck with a combination stretch and lifting movement. An advantage of this exercise is that it can be done in either the standing or reclining position depending on the individual's preference.

## Technique

1. Lie or stand in a relaxed position with the arms to the sides of the body. If lying on the ground, lift the shoulders sufficiently to clear the ground when the head is in its maximum rearward position.

2. Moving in a clockwise direction, first tilt the head toward the right shoulder, holding it for a single count at its point of maximum lateral flexion. (Count 1)

3. Tilt the head back from the right shoulder, extending the chin up from the chest. Hold the head back at its point of maximum extension for a single count. (Count 2)

4. Continuing to move in a clockwise direction, tilt the head forward and to the side, toward the left shoulder. Hold the head for a single count at its point of maximum lateral flexion toward the left shoulder. (Count 3)

5. Tilt the head forward from the left shoulder, lowering the chin to the chest. Hold the head forward with the chin against the chest for a single count. (Count 4)

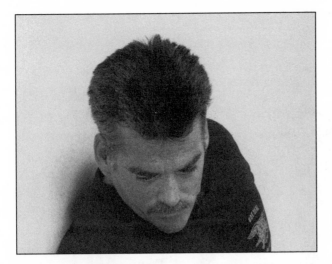
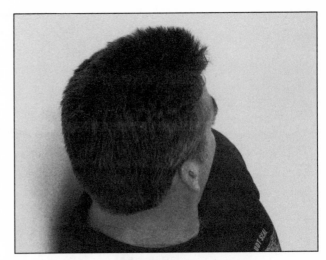
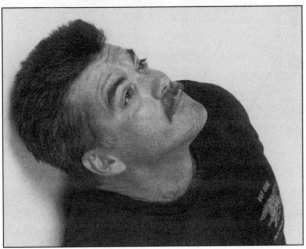
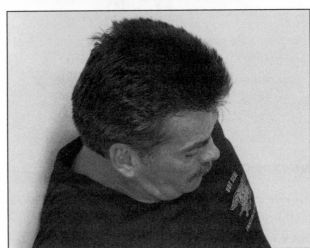

**Repetition.** The above completes a single repetition of a four-count, clockwise neck rotation. A complete set of neck rotations includes both clockwise and counterclockwise movements.

**Advantages.** This is a very light exercise for loosening and building up the neck muscles. Though it can be done in both the standing and reclining position, it is most often done in the Teams in the reclining position.

**Disadvantages.** Care must be taken not to strike the head against the ground when doing this exercise in the reclining position.

WARNINGS. Do not force resistance against the neck while doing this exercise by pushing against the head with the hands. Make certain the upper body is held sufficiently clear of the ground to prevent striking the head. Do not hyperextend the neck, tilting the head backward past the midline of the body, as you could injure the neck or spine.

*Note.* This exercise can also be done as a two-count movement by tilting the head forward only to the chin and extending it backward. This movement is called a fore-and-aft neck rotation.

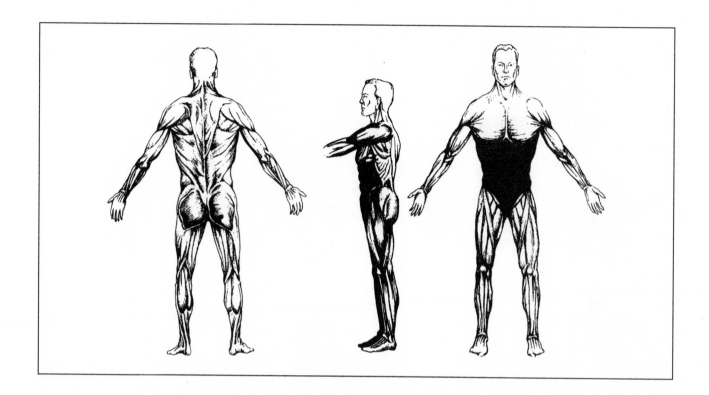

## ABDOMINAL EXERCISES

### STANDARD SIT-UP

**Muscle groups.** Abdominals, primarily the rectus abdominis, and external and internal obliques.

A very basic exercise, the sit-up has been modified within the last few years due to studies done on the musculature involved. The standard sit-up, also called the bent leg sit-up, is used as a measure of abdominal strength, judged by the number of sit-ups that can be properly performed in a set amount of time.

### Technique

1. Lying flat on the back, flex the knees at a 45-degree angle. The feet are held flat to the floor and close together. The arms are crossed on the chest, hands underneath the armpits, and the elbows close to the body. Keep the head held straight and the eyes looking forward throughout the movements.

*Note.* If the legs lift during the exercise, place the feet underneath a heavy object such as a piece of furniture. If such an object is not available, extend the legs out to a 90-degree angle at the knees and continue.

2. Lift the upper body smoothly to the sitting position without putting the elbows forward from either arm position. Roll the spine up to a sitting position by pulling the weight up with the abdominal muscles. Stop when the forearms touch the knees or thighs. (Count 1)

3. Lower the upper body back to the starting position in a slow, controlled movement. (Count 2)

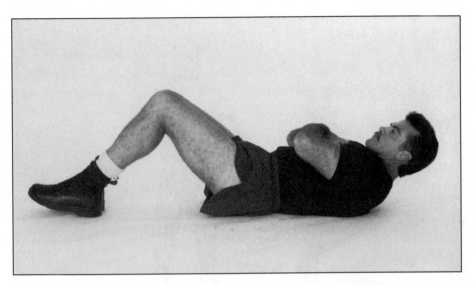

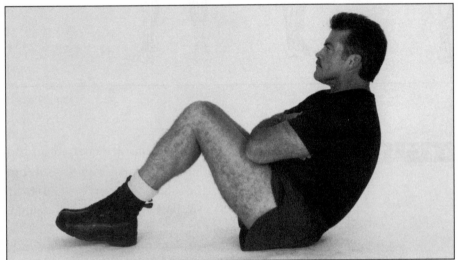

**Repetition.** The above completes one repetition of a two-count sit-up.

**Advantages.** This is a strong and simple, basic exercise for building up the major abdominal muscles.

**Disadvantages.** The lower back is easily injured in this exercise if the movement is uncontrolled or the workout surface too hard. Do not lace the fingers behind the head in the old style and pull forward as that action may injure the neck. The

elbows and arms need to be held close to the chest while in the starting position and not jerked forward to build up momentum.

WARNINGS. This exercise puts the lower back at a high risk of injury. Keep the movement smooth and controlled, maintaining a rounded contour to the lower back through the full range of motions. Do not clasp the hands behind the neck or head as this may cause neck injuries by forcing the head too far forward.

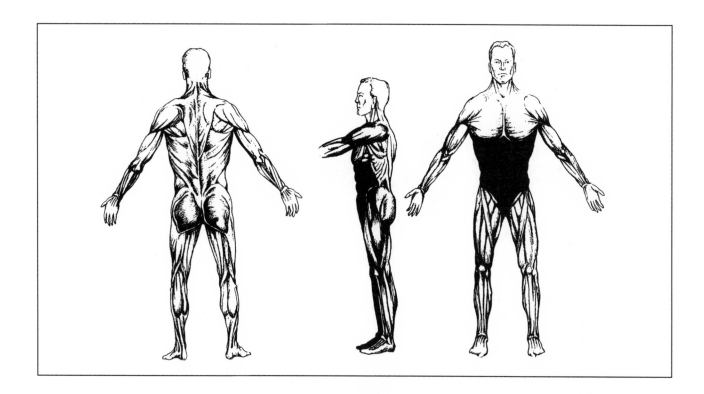

## HALF SIT-UPS

**Muscle groups.** Abdominals, primarily the rectus abdominis, and external and internal obliques.

This exercise concentrates the effort to complete the movement on both the main upper and lower muscles of the abdomen.

### Technique

1. Lying flat on the back, flex the knees at a 90-degree angle. Hold the feet flat to the floor and close together, with the hands placed lightly on the hips, thumbs along the sides, and fingers pointing toward the center of the stomach. Keep the head held straight and looking forward throughout the movements.

2. Lift the upper body smoothly halfway up to the sitting position without putting the elbows forward from either arm position. Roll the spine up to a sitting position by pulling the weight up with the abdominal muscles. Stop when the body is raised halfway and the torso is at a 45-degree angle to the floor. (Count 1)

*Note.* The exercise is made harder by holding the torso in the raised position for a count of ten. This paused exercise is used as part of a normal set of repetitions. A suggestion would be to make the last five repetitions of a twenty-count set paused half sit-ups.

3. Lower the upper body back to the starting position in a slow, controlled movement. (Count 2)

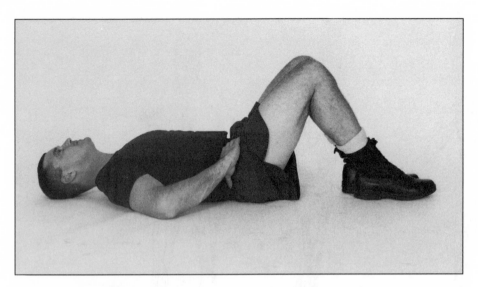

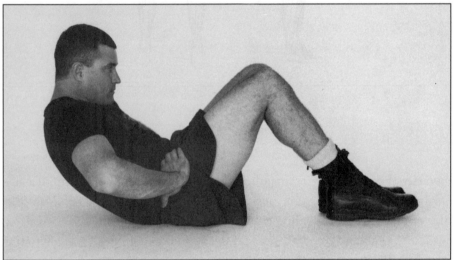

**Repetition.** The above completes one repetition of a two-count half sit-up.

**Advantages.** This is a strong and simple, basic exercise for building up the major abdominal muscles. Adding a pause to the first count of the movement greatly increases the potential value of the exercise.

**Disadvantages.** The lower back is easily injured in this exercise if the movement is uncontrolled or the workout surface too hard. The elbows and arms need to be held in the starting position and not jerked forward to build up momentum.

WARNINGS. This exercise puts the lower back at a high risk of injury or strain. Keep the movement smooth and controlled, maintaining a rounded contour to the lower back through the full range of motions.

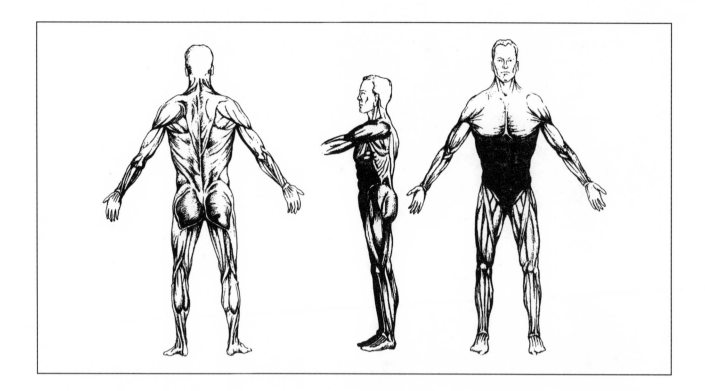

## CROSS-LEG SIT-UPS, RIGHT/LEFT (CROSSOVERS)

**Muscle groups.** Abdominals, primarily the external and internal obliques and the rectus abdominis.

This variation of the sit-up concentrates the effort of the movement on the oblique muscles as well as the primary abdominals. The mechanics of this exercise combine those of the sit-up and the crunch with a twisting action added to increase the effort of the oblique muscles.

### Technique

1. While lying flat on the back, bend the left leg at a 45-degree angle with the sole of the left foot flat on the floor. Then bend the right leg and bring it across the left leg with the right ankle braced behind the left knee, making a triangle. The right arm is extended down along the right side of the body and lies, palm down, flat on the floor. The left arm is raised above the shoulder, bent at the elbow, and the left hand lightly cups the left ear.

2. Without pulling the head up, move the left arm across the body until the elbow touches the upper right leg, as close to the knee as possible. Bend and lift the upper body as needed to reach the leg. Keep the lower back pressed against the floor and maintain the tension of the abdominal muscles during the entire movement of the exercise. (Count 1)

3. Lower the left arm and body in a smooth, controlled movement, not allowing the left shoulder to contact the ground. (Count 2)

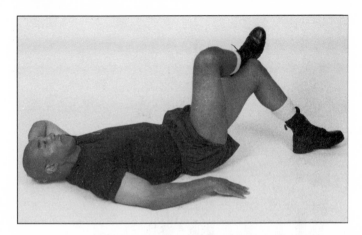

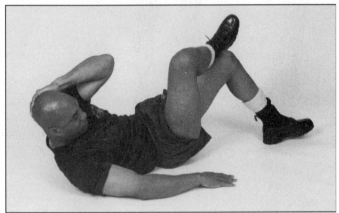

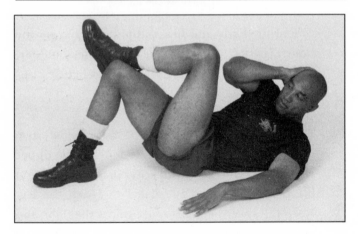

**Repetition.** The above completes a single repetition of a two-count left cross-leg sit-up.

For a right cross-leg sit-up, repeat the above technique reversing the arms and legs. Continue with the right cross-leg sit-ups after completing the full set of left-side exercises.

**Advantages.** This exercise works the upper and lower oblique muscles fully while still involving the other muscles of the abdomen. The minimum movement of the lower back limits the risk of damage to the back.

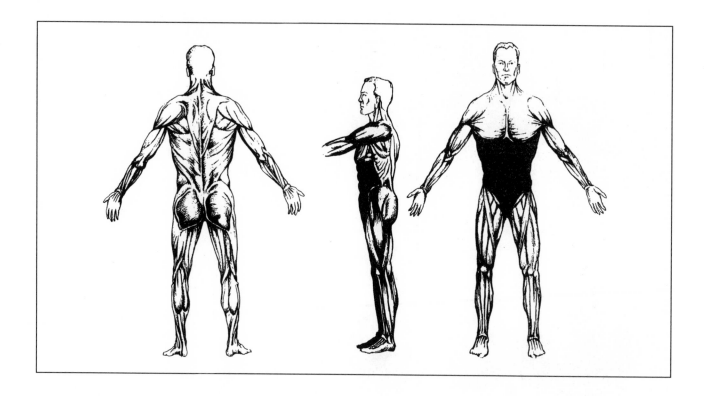

## EXTENDED LEG CRUNCHES

**Muscle groups.** Abdominals, especially the upper rectus abdominis as well as the upper and lower obliques.

This exercise gives a heavy workout to the abdominal muscles utilizing a relatively small movement of the body.

### Technique

1. Lie flat on the floor with the legs extended out, feet together and toes pointed up. Lifting the arms above the shoulders, put the fingers behind the head and hold the elbows flat to the floor.

2. While holding the elbows and arms back, lift the head, shoulders, and upper back up, curling forward with the upper portion of the abdominal muscle. Raise up until the chin is touching the chest and the upper back and the lower portion of the shoulder blades is just clear of the floor. DO NOT pull the head forward with the hands. Hold in the up position for a second or two while also squeezing the abdominal muscles. (Count 1)

3. Slowly lower the upper body and head back to the starting position, straightening the neck and raising the chin. Do not rest the shoulders or head on the floor when in the down position. (Count 2)

*Note.* The arms may also be held crossed in front of the chest. When using the crossed-arm posture, do not raise the arms from the chest in order to "pull" the upper body forward. To increase the impact of this exercise, a weight may be held in the arms when using the crossed-arm posture.

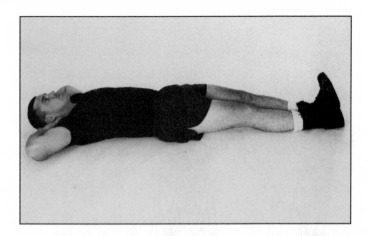

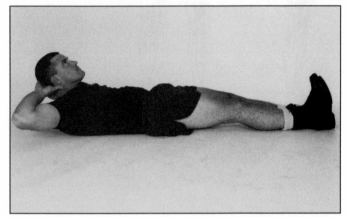

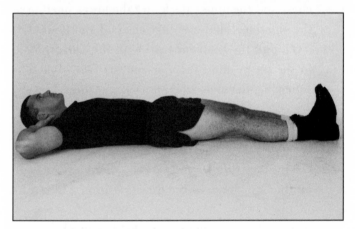

**Repetition.** The above completes a single repetition of a two-count extended leg crunch.

**Advantages.** This exercise is as effective as or more effective than—and has a much lower risk to the lower back—a number of older calisthenic movements that are now discouraged.

**Disadvantages.** The hands-behind-the-head posture can lead the individual to pull the head forward during the exercise.

WARNINGS. Do not pull forward on the head with the hands while doing this exercise. Neck injuries can result from forcing (hyperextending) the head forward.

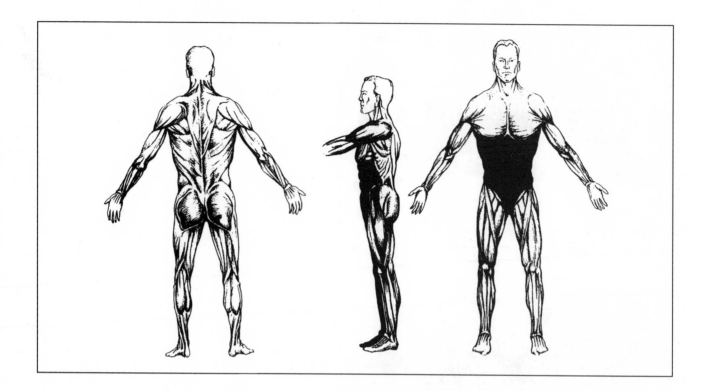

## BENT LEG CRUNCHES

**Muscle groups.** Abdominals, especially the upper rectus abdominis as well as the upper and lower obliques.

This exercise gives a more intense workout to the abdominal muscles while still utilizing a relatively small movement of the body.

## Technique

1. While lying flat on the floor, bend at the knees, bringing the feet in toward the buttocks, keeping the soles of the feet flat on the floor. Bring the legs in as tightly as possible while still keeping the feet flat on the floor. Lifting the arms above the shoulders, put the fingers behind the head and hold the elbows flat to the floor.

2. While holding the elbows and arms back, lift up the head, shoulders, and upper back, curling forward with the upper portion of the abdominal muscle. Raise up until the chin is touching the chest and the upper back and the lower portion of the shoulder blades is just clear of the floor. DO NOT pull the head forward with the hands. Hold in the up position for a second or two while also squeezing the abdominal muscles. (Count 1)

3. Slowly lower the upper body and head back to the starting position, straightening the neck and raising the chin. Do not rest the shoulders or head on the floor when in the down position. (Count 2)

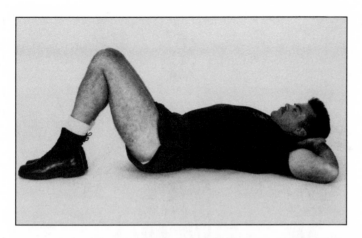

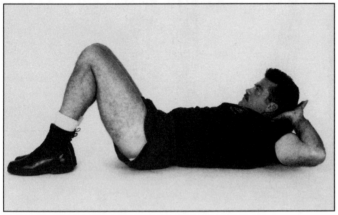

**Repetition.** The above completes a single repetition of a two-count bent leg crunch.

**Advantages.** This is a very effective exercise for working the abdominal muscles at a very low risk to the lower back.

**Disadvantages.** The hands behind the head posture can lead the individual to pull the head forward during the exercise.

WARNINGS. Do not pull forward on the head with the hands while doing this exercise. Neck injuries can result from forcing (hyperextending) the head forward.

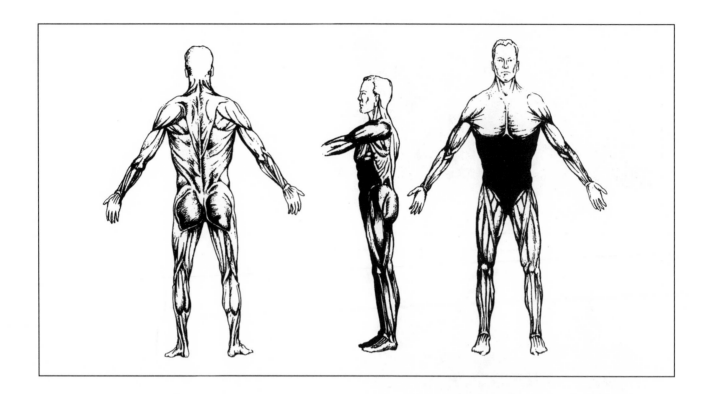

## RAISED BENT LEG CRUNCHES

**Muscle groups.** Abdominals, especially the upper rectus abdominis and the upper and lower obliques.

This exercise gives an intense workout to the abdominal muscles, including the obliques, with only a small movement of the body.

### Technique

1. While flat on the floor, raise the legs to a 90-degree angle with the waist while bending at the knees to a comfortable position. Crossing the ankles helps stabilize the position of the legs. Lifting the arms above the shoulders, put the fingers behind the head, holding the elbows straight out to the sides.

2. Bending the arms to put the elbows forward, lift the head, shoulders, and upper back up, curling forward with the upper portion of the abdominal muscle. Raise up until elbows touch the upper legs. DO NOT pull the head forward with the hands. Hold in the up position for a second or two while also squeezing the abdominal muscles. (Count 1)

3. Slowly lower the upper body and head back to the starting position, straightening the neck, raising the chin, and putting the elbows back out to the sides. Do not rest the shoulders or head on the floor when in the down position. (Count 2)

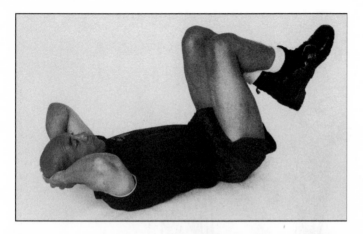

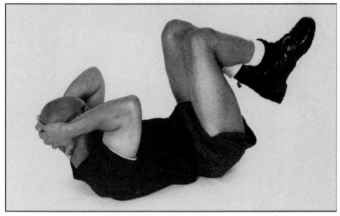

**Repetition.** The above completes a single repetition of a two-count raised bent leg crunch.

**Advantages.** This is one of the most intense workouts given to the abdominal muscles by a crunch-type exercise. There is little risk to the lower back during this movement.

**Disadvantages.** It is particularly easy to pull forward on the head while doing this exercise.

WARNINGS. Be very careful not to pull forward on the head while doing this exercise. Do not lace the fingers behind the head but hold the back of the head gently with the fingers spread.

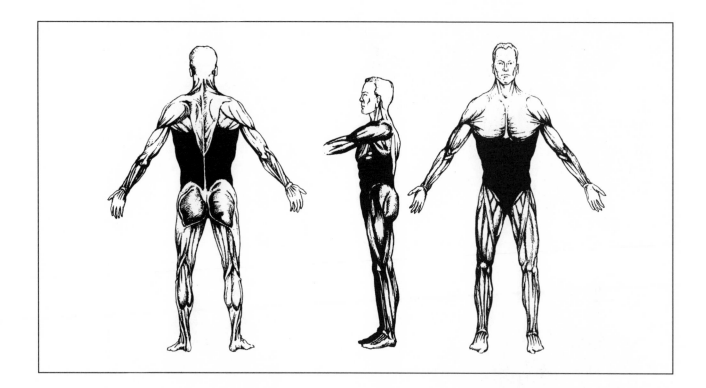

## TRUNK ROTATIONS

**Muscle groups.** Abdomen and lower back, including the rectus abdominis, internal and external obliques, the latissimus dorsi, lumbodorsal fascia, and sacrospinalis.

This exercise is a more active version of the trunk stretch. Working the muscles around the entire abdomen, this movement particularly stretches and builds up the lower-back muscles at a gradual rate.

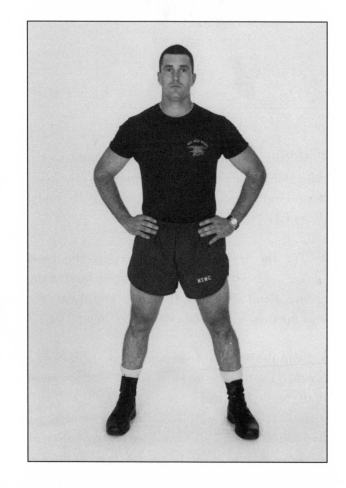

### Technique

1. Stand straight with the feet shoulder-width apart, bending the elbows outward. Put the hands lightly on the hips, fingers forward, thumbs toward the back. Keep the eyes looking straight ahead.

2. Bend forward at the waist as far as you are able, keeping the head square on the shoulders and the eyes facing the floor. (Count 1)

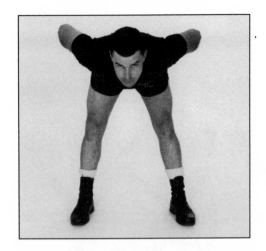

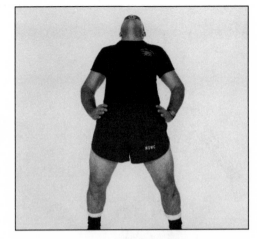

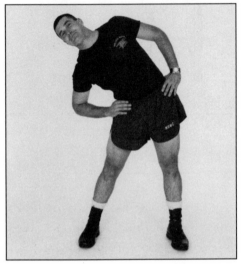

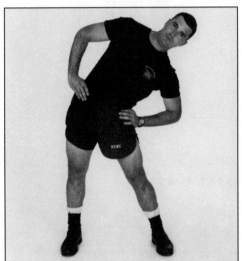

3. Moving in a clockwise direction, bend to the right side as far as possible, keeping the eyes looking forward and the arms square to the body. (Count 2)

4. Tilt the body backward, keeping the head square to the shoulders and looking up toward the ceiling. Bend slightly at the knees and thrust the hips forward to maintain balance. (Count 3)

5. Bend to the left side as much as possible, keeping the eyes looking forward and the arms square to the body. (Count 4)

**Repetition.** The above completes one repetition of a four-count clockwise trunk rotation. Half of a

set of trunk rotations are made in a clockwise direction. The remainder of the set are made in a counterclockwise direction.

**Advantages.** A very low-impact exercise that helps build up the back muscles as well as maintain the flexibility of all the trunk muscles.

**Disadvantages.** Bending too far to the rear can compress disks in the back and otherwise injure it.

WARNINGS. To prevent hyperextending and possibly injuring the back when bending to the rear, keep the knees bent slightly.

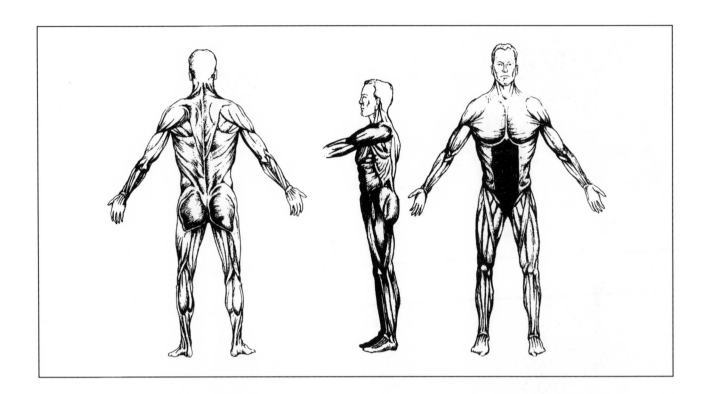

## HIP THRUST (PELVIC TILT)

**Muscle groups.** Both upper and lower portions of the rectus abdominis.

This is a very low-impact exercise that only involves the abdominal muscles when done correctly.

### Technique

1. While lying flat on the floor, bend at the knees to pull the feet up toward the buttocks. Keep the soles of the feet flat on the floor and try to pull the leg to a 45-degree angle or less. Place the hands in a comfortable position on the stomach or to the sides.

2. Rotate the pelvis up and back toward the rib cage by contracting the abdominal muscles. Keep the small of the back pushed down into the floor. Do not lift the buttocks from the floor with the legs; rather, rotate the hips with the abdomen. When the pelvis is rotated to its maximum, hold it in position for two seconds. (Count 1)

3. Rotate the pelvis smoothly back to its starting position, allowing the small of the back to move up off the floor slightly. (Count 2)

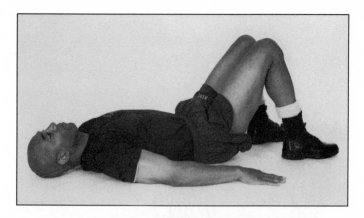

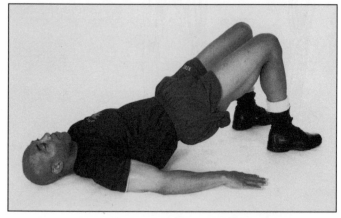

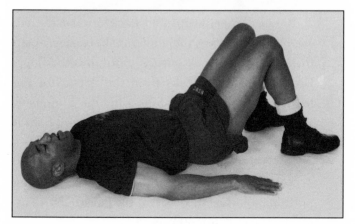

**Repetition.** The above completes a single repetition of a two-count hip thrust.

**Advantages.** This exercise builds up the abdominal muscles with very little risk to the lower back.

**Disadvantages.** A subtle exercise with a very slow buildup of the abdominal muscles.

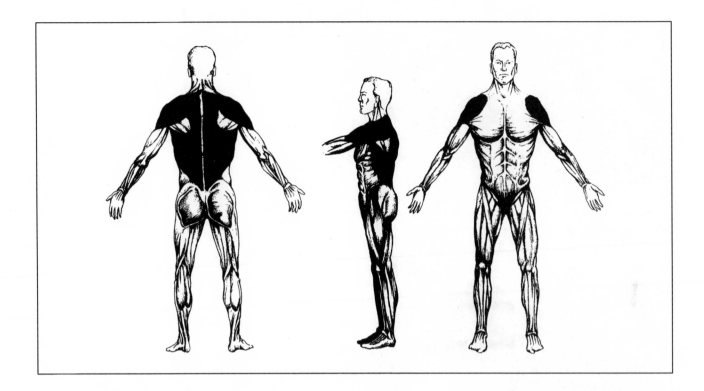

## WAVE-OFFS

**Muscle groups.** Shoulders and upper back, particularly the trapezius, deltoid, and latissimus dorsi.

Resembling a skydiving position, this exercise builds up both the strength and flexibility of the shoulders. The lower back is also strengthened from holding the position.

### Technique

1. While lying on the stomach, bend the knees and raise the lower legs straight up into the air. The legs should be spaced slightly apart for stability. Arch the back and lift the head and upper chest up off the floor. With the arms held about 6 inches above the floor, bend the elbows to a 90-degree angle, crossing the hands about a foot or so in front of the face. The hands are held palms down and crossed with the fingers of one hand above those of the other.

2. With the eyes looking forward and the chest, shoulders, and arms above the floor, sweep the arms out to the sides and back as far as possible, straightening the bend in the elbows as necessary. (Count 1)

3. Sweep the arms forward again, bending at the elbows. Return to the starting position with the hands crossed one above the other in front of the face. (Count 2)

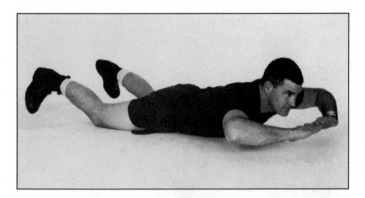

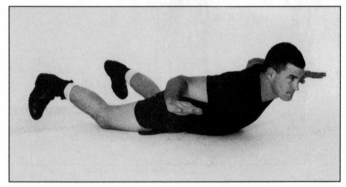

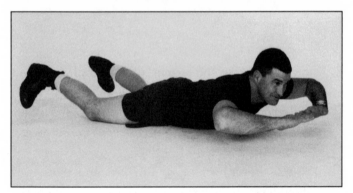

**Repetition.** The above completes one repetition of a two-count wave-off.

**Advantages.** This exercise builds up the flexibility and strength in the shoulder muscles as well as having a lesser effect on the muscles of the lower back.

WARNINGS. Do not hyperextend the neck when raising the head back. Hold the head in a comfortable up position.

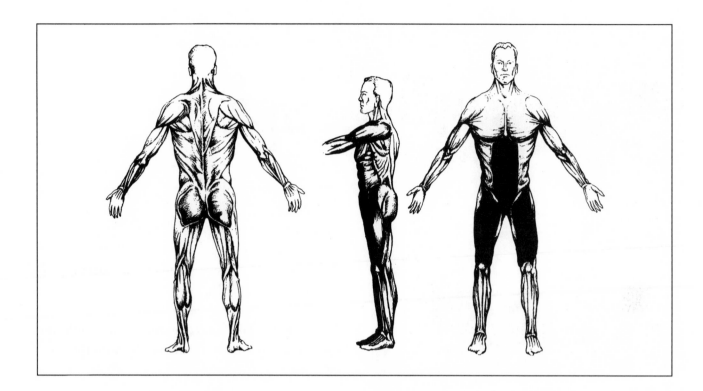

## LEG LEVERS

**Muscle groups.** Abdominals and upper legs, specifically the rectus abdominis and quadriceps femoris.

This exercise uses much of the movement of the knee bend but eliminates strain on the knees and lower back by limiting the amount of weight lifted to just that of the legs.

### Technique

1. Begin lying flat on the back with the arms straight and the hands placed underneath the buttocks. The legs are extended straight out with a slight bend at the knees and are together with the feet square and the toes pointed up. The legs are raised so that the heels are 6 inches above the floor. The head is raised up off of the floor with the chin down toward the chest.

2. The legs are raised until the heels are several feet off the floor and the legs are between a 45- and 90-degree angle to the floor. (Count 1)

3. The legs are lowered smoothly and held up when the heels are again 6 inches from the floor. (Count 2)

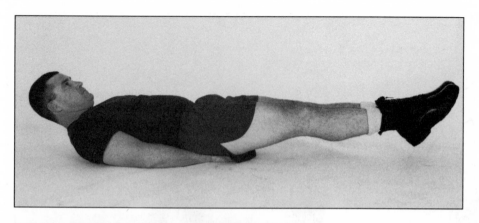

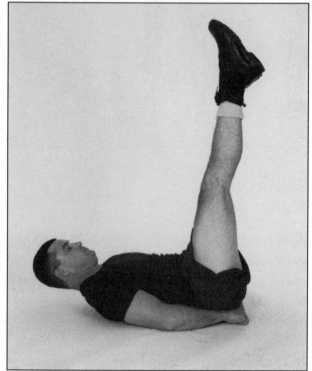

**Repetition.** The above completes a single repetition of a two-count leg lever.

**Advantages.** This exercise builds up both the abdominal and upper thigh muscles with the same movement.

**Disadvantages.** This exercise can put a heavy strain on the lower back. Keep a slight bend in the knees throughout the movement to minimize muscle strain. Beginning users may try raising only one leg at a time until the muscles have built up for the full movement.

WARNING. Immediately cease the exercise if any serious pulling or pain is felt in the lower back.

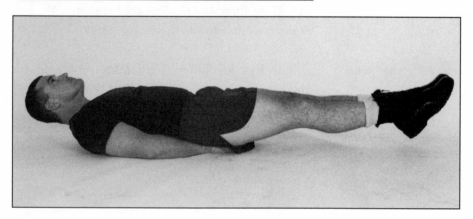

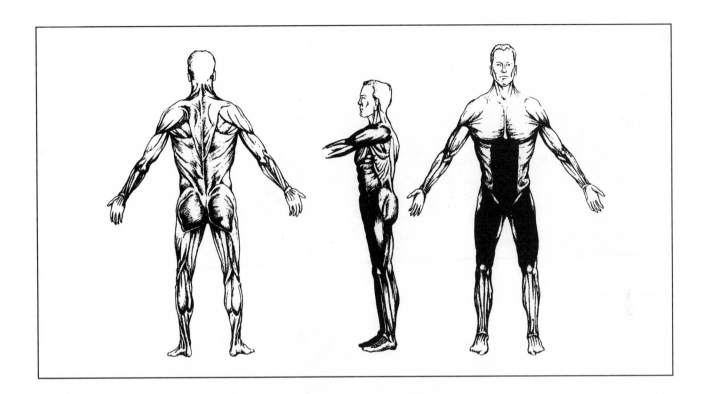

## KNEE-UPS

**Muscle groups.** Abdominals and upper legs, specifically the rectus abdominis and quadriceps femoris.

This exercise works the muscles of the abdomen and upper thighs at a much lower risk to the lower back.

## Technique

1. Lie flat on the back in a relaxed position with the arms angled out from the sides and the palms down on the floor. Put the soles of the feet flat on the floor and move the heels in toward the buttocks until the knees are at a 45-degree angle or less.

2. Bring the knees up toward the chest, rolling up on the lower back. Raise the buttocks and lower back up off the floor until the knees touch the chest. (Count 1)

3. Lower the feet back to the floor slowly, rolling the back down smoothly and slowly. (Count 2)

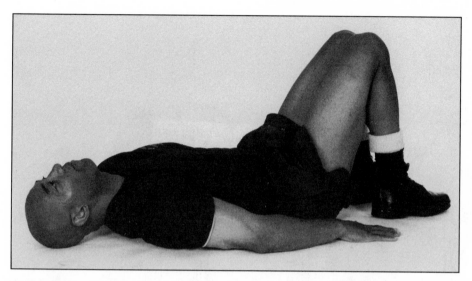

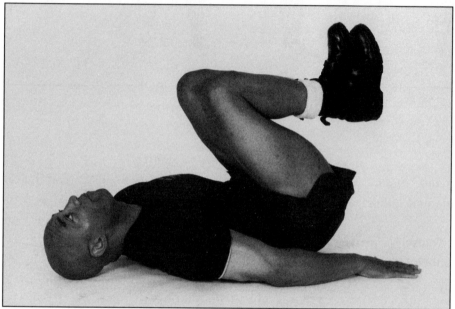

**Repetition.** The above completes one repetition of a two-count knee-up.

**Advantages.** This exercise fully contracts the lower abdominal muscles while still keeping the back at a low risk of strain.

**Disadvantages.** Initial movements done with this exercise may be limited until greater flexibility is developed in the back and legs.

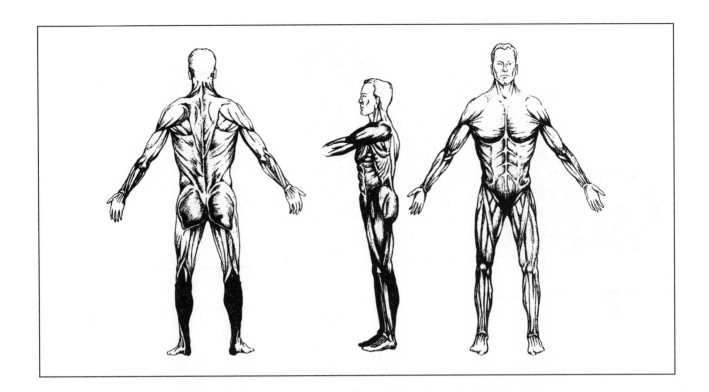

## CALF RAISES

**Muscle groups.** Lower legs, particularly the gastrocnemius, soleus, and plantaris muscles as well as the achilles tendon.

This is a low-impact exercise that concentrates its action almost fully on the targeted muscles. The two variations of the exercise allow for an easy increase in effect.

### Technique (Two-Legged)

1. Standing with the legs straight and the feet about shoulder-width apart, rest the hands lightly on the hips.

2. Lift the heels of both feet simultaneously by flexing down on the balls of the feet. The pace is moderate with the lift taking one or two seconds. (Count 1)

3. Lower the heels in a smooth, controlled manner with the full movement done over a period of one or two seconds. (Count 2)

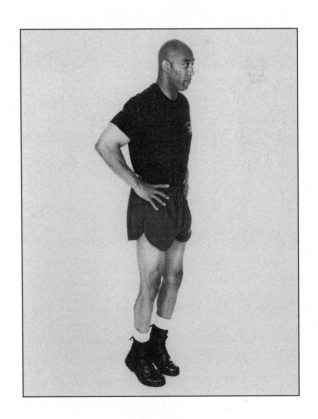

**Repetition.** The above completes one repetition of a two-count two-legged calf raise.

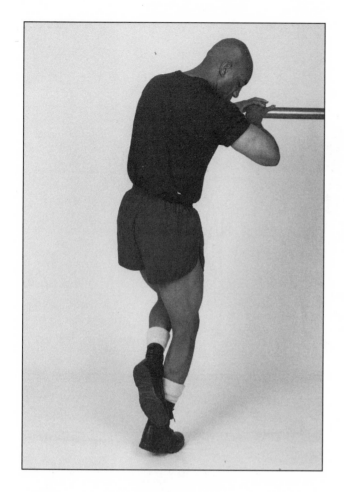
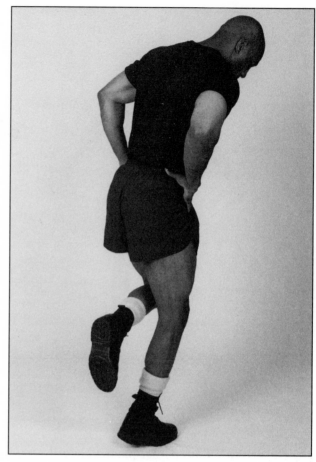

## Technique (One-Legged)

1. While holding on to a solid object for stability, hook the left foot around the back of the right ankle. The body is held straight and any free hand is placed lightly on the hip.

2. The heel of the right foot is raised several inches by flexing down with the ball of the foot. The lift of the body is done at a moderate pace over a second or two. (Count 1)

3. The right foot is relaxed and lowered to bring the body down in a smooth, controlled manner at the same pace as the initial lift. (Count 2)

**Repetition.** The above completes one repetition of a two-count one-legged calf raise. After half of the set is completed with the right foot, the remaining repetitions are done with the left foot.

**Advantages.** The two-legged calf raise is the more stable exercise. The spread legs help to keep balance during the movement, and the weight of the body is divided between the calves making the overall exercise easier. The one-legged calf raise is a more intense exercise for the more advanced individual.

**Disadvantages.** The one-legged calf raise is an unstable position. To prevent a possible loss of balance, a sturdy support is suggested.

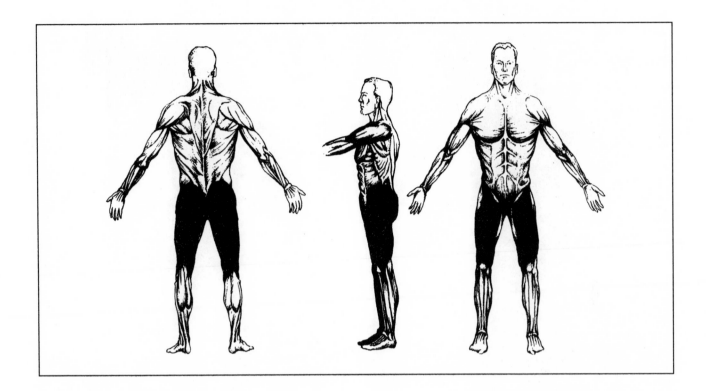

## LUNGES

**Muscle groups.** Upper and lower leg, buttocks, and lower back, particularly the quadriceps femoris, gluteus maximus, and hamstrings.

This exercise works the entire leg and buttocks area with particular emphasis on the front and back of the thighs. This basic movement has a number of variations available.

## Technique

1. The body is standing straight with the feet shoulder width or less apart. The hands are resting lightly on the hips, thumbs on the belt line with the fingers facing toward the front center. The elbows are bent and sticking out to the sides. The back and neck are held aligned throughout the movement with the head straight and the eyes looking forward.

2. Stepping out with the left foot first, keep the right foot in place. Make the size of the step long enough so that when the knee is bent it will not extend past the toe of the forward foot. Keep the shin square to the ground. Continuing forward with the movement, keep the body upright while lowering the right knee to just touch the ground. (Count 1)

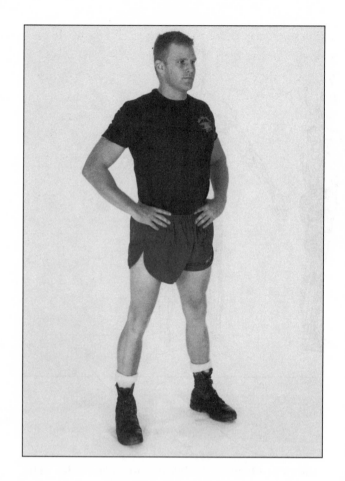

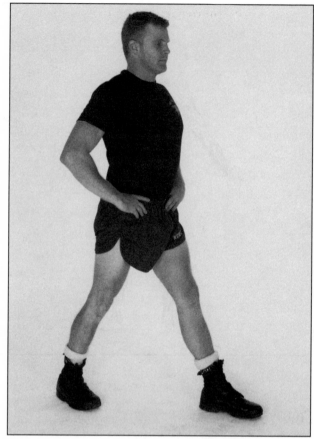

3. Pushing back with the left leg, bring the body back up. Continuing the movement, draw the left foot smoothly back to the starting position. (Count 2)

4. The movement is continued by stepping out with the right foot and bringing the left knee down to lightly touch the ground. (Count 3)

5. Pushing back with the right foot, bring the body back to an up position and draw the right foot back to the starting position in a single, smooth movement. (Count 4)

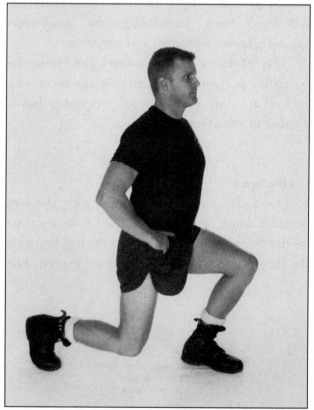

**Repetition.** The above completes one repetition of a four-count lunge.

**Advantages.** This exercise strongly works the entire lower body. More benefit is received from the movement by raising up from the down position forcefully and quickly. A method of building up the value of the exercise is to add weight to the body. A standard barbell, with a low beginning weight, can be held across the front of the chest or on the shoulders behind the neck. Dumbbells can also be held in the hands with the arms hanging down during the movement to add weight.

**Disadvantages.** The body must be held in a straight position, with the neck and spine in line, throughout the exercise. Bending forward while doing the movement puts excessive strain on the lower back. Spreading the feet farther apart can aid in keeping balance. Care must be taken when using a barbell and adding weight that it is not too heavy. Particular care must be taken that a barbell does not strike or ride on the back of the neck during the movement.

WARNINGS. Do not rise too forcefully as this can overstrain the front muscles of the lead leg.

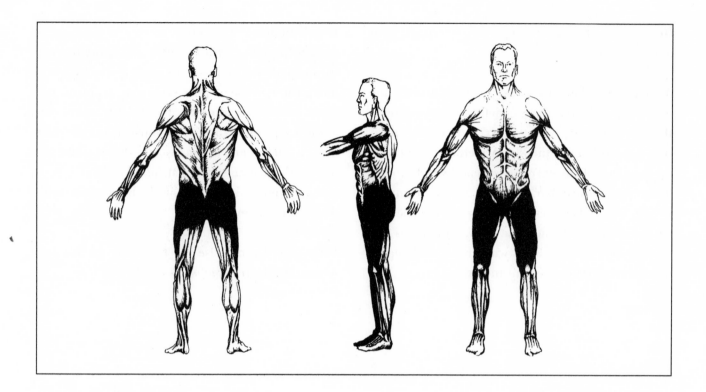

## STAR JUMPERS

**Muscle groups.** Legs, especially the quadriceps femoris and gluteus maximus.

This exercise helps to build explosive power in the legs, a combination of both speed and strength.

### Technique
1. With the feet shoulder-width apart, bend the legs and lower the body into a crouching position until the knees are at a 90-degree angle. Bend the arms at the elbows and hold them at the sides with the hands in an open position.

2. The arms are first swung back and then forward and up above the shoulders. As the arms swing forward, the legs are straightened and the body vigorously jumps into the air. The swing of the arms is continued through the jump and they are stretched above the shoulders, reaching up with spread fingers. (Count 1)

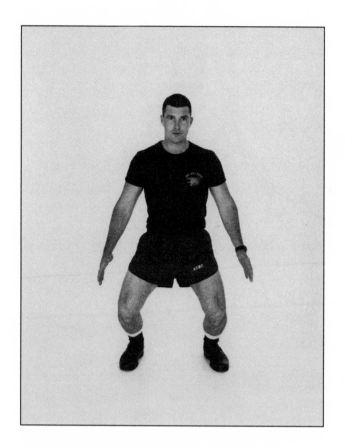
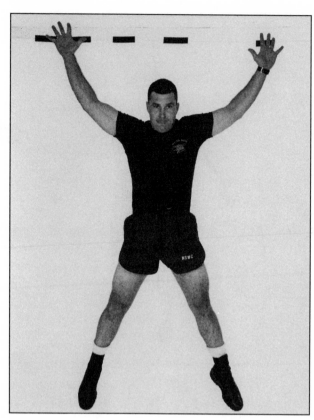

3. As the body comes back down, it recovers in the crouching position with the arms bent. (Count 2)

4. Continue with the repetitions, moving the arms in a smooth arc throughout the movement.

**Repetition.** The above completes one repetition of the two-count star jumper.

**Advantages.** This exercise combines a muscle-building movement with a stretch. Coordination and balance are also increased.

**Disadvantages.** This is very hard to conduct indoors in a normal dwelling. Make sure there is sufficient overhead clearance.

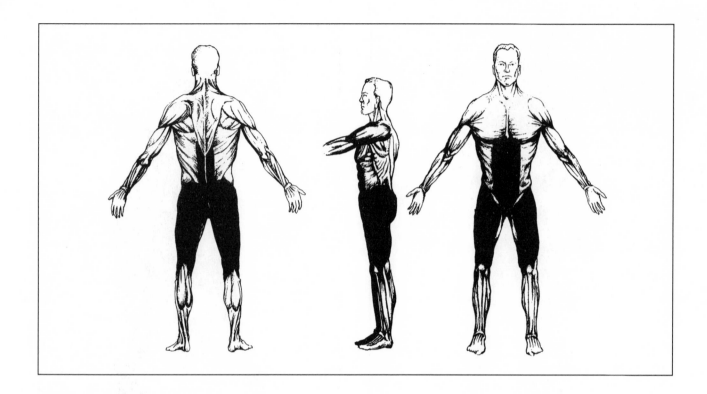

## HALF-DEEP KNEE BEND (TOUCH YOUR BOOTS)

**Muscle groups.** Upper legs, lower back, and abdominal muscles, especially the quadriceps femoris, hamstrings, gluteus maximus, rectus abdominis, lumbodorsal fascia, and sacrospinalis.

This is the safest version of the knee bend series of exercises and is the calisthenic version of the free-weight squat. By only lowering the body a short distance, stress on the knees is kept at a minimum.

### Technique

1. Starting with the feet shoulder-width apart, hold the back straight with the neck and keep the head facing forward. The arms are out to the sides with the hands resting on the hips.

2. While keeping the eyes looking forward and the back straight, bend the knees to lower the body. At the same time, the hands come off the hips and reach straight down to the full extent of the arms. The knees are bent until the hands can slap the top of the boots or socks (mid-calf) on the outside of the legs. (Count 1)

3. After touching the boot tops, raise the body smoothly, placing the hands back on the hips. (Count 2)

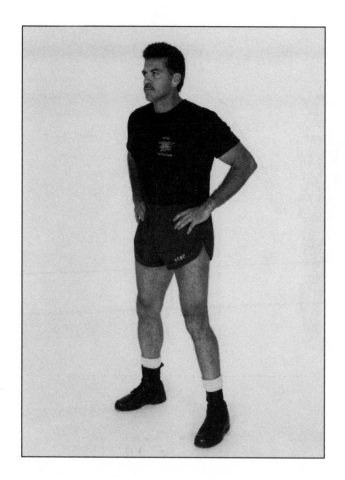

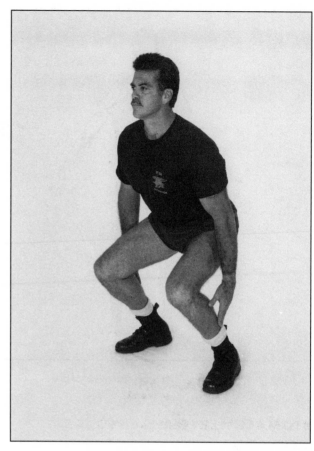

**Repetition.** This completes one repetition of a two-count half-deep knee bend.

**Advantages.** This exercise is considered one of the best calisthenic movements available for the legs. The raising movement can be done at a quicker pace than the squat for greater benefit. Not going too deep into the knee bend means that the ligaments of the knee are not stretched to any great extent.

**Disadvantages.** Going too deep and bouncing at the bottom of the squat can damage the knee ligaments.

WARNINGS. Do not squat past the point where the knees bend 90 degrees. Keep the back straight to minimize strain on the lower back.

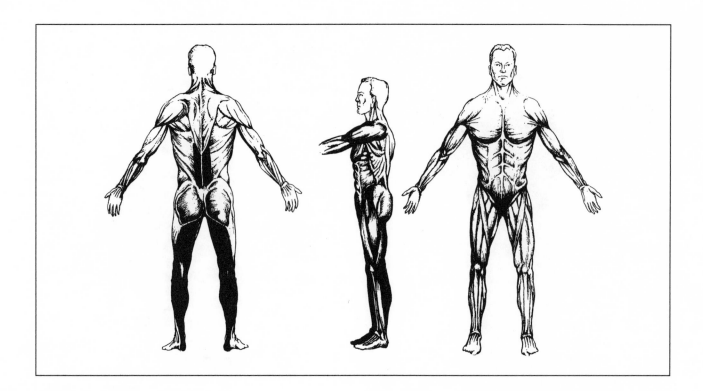

## STOMACH FLUTTER KICKS

**Muscle groups.** Calves, lower back, and rear thighs, especially the gastrocnemius, soleus, and plantaris muscles, the hamstrings, and the lumbodorsal fascia and sacrospinalis muscles.

This movement most closely duplicates the motions of an underwater swimmer. The actions of this exercise build up the leg muscles used by a SEAL while swimming. This is the last of the flutter kick exercises still used to build up a specific portion of the body.

### Technique

1. Lying flat on the stomach, move the hands and arms above the shoulders. The elbows are straightened past a 90-degree angle and the hands are spaced greater than shoulder-width apart.

The legs are stretched out with the feet shoulder-width apart and the toes pointed out to the rear. Raise the arms, legs, and upper chest, clear of the floor, so that the arms and legs are a foot or more off the floor. The head is kept up and the eyes look straight ahead.

2. Raise the right leg higher into the air while simultaneously lowering the left leg an equal distance. Keep the feet extended and the toes pointing to the rear. The legs should be kept straight and the arms are allowed to move in the opposite direction of the legs if desired or held still. (Count 1)

3. Reverse the motion, lowering the right leg and raising the left. (Count 2)

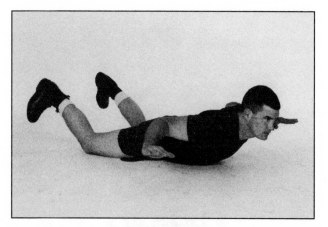

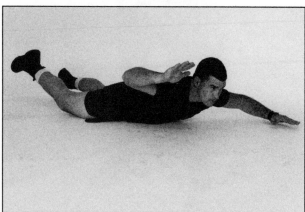

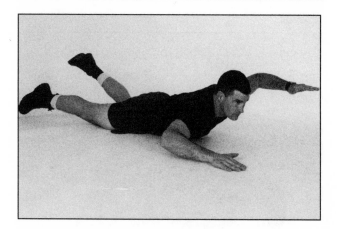

**Disadvantages.** A difficult exercise to complete properly until the muscles build up.

WARNINGS. Do not strain the muscles attempting this exercise. Do not force yourself to complete the full set but do what you are able to with no great strain to the body.

**Repetition.** The above completes one repetition of a two-count flutter kick.

**Advantages.** This exercise builds up the muscles needed for swimming underwater, especially with fins.

## GENERAL

### EIGHT-COUNT BODY BUILDERS

**Muscle groups.** All the major muscle groups of the body are worked in this exercise.

This exercise combines the movements of a number of separate exercises. It is particularly strenuous as it works the legs, arms, shoulders, abdominals, back, and chest muscles in a series of motions.

### Technique

1. Begin in the standing position with the legs straight, feet shoulder-width apart, and the head facing forward. Place the hands on the hips with the elbows bent out to the sides.

2. Bend forward, putting the arms straight down. Bend the knees until the hands touch the floor, shoulder-width apart. (Count 1)

3. Bouncing up with the feet, snap the legs back while still in the air. Land on the toes with the feet together and the legs fully extended. This is the starting position for the push-up. (Count 2)

4. Lower your body to the floor by bending the elbows and rotating the shoulders. Keep the legs and back straight during all phases of this movement. Stop lowering your body when your chest lightly touches the floor. (Count 3)

5. Push the upper body back up to the starting position with a smooth motion, keeping the legs and back straight. (Count 4)

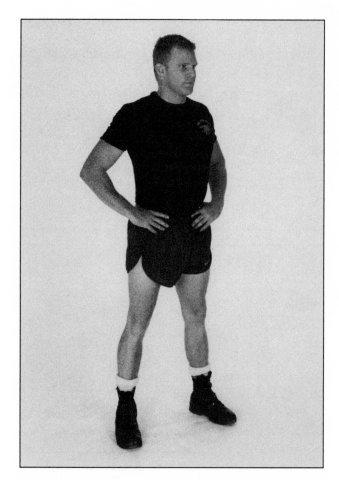

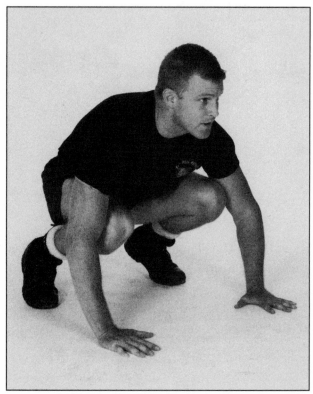

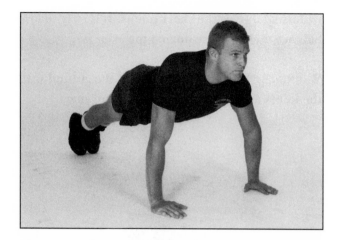

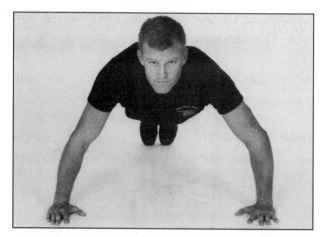

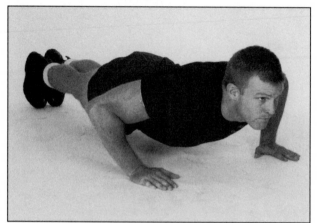

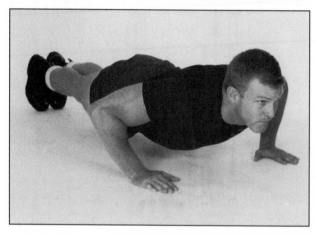

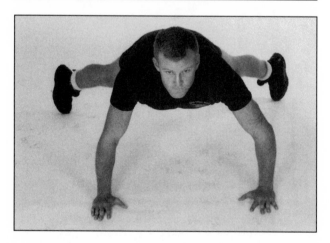

6. From the push-up position, spring up with the legs. While the legs are still in the air, spread them to a 45-degree angle and land on the toes. Keep the back and legs straight and the head up and looking forward. (Count 5)

7. From the legs-spread position, again spring up with the legs. With the feet off the ground, snap the legs back together. Land in the push-up position. (Count 6)

8. Jump up with the toes, keeping the hands on the ground, and draw the knees in to the body. Land in the crouching position from Count 1 with the feet together. (Count 7)

9. Raise up from the crouching position, lifting with the legs. Stand upright with the hands on the hips and the elbows extended out to the sides. (Count 8)

**Repetition.** The above completes one repetition of an eight-count body builder.

**Advantages.** This exercise works the entire body and is one of the more strenuous movements.

**Disadvantages.** The exercise cannot be done without sufficient strength in the legs to move them

with snap during the short jumps. It is easy to lose balance and collapse during the exercise.

WARNINGS. Take care not to strike the ground with the knees at any point during the movement.

# FREE WEIGHT TRAINING

THE USE OF free weights is the most common form of isotonic training after calisthenics. Instead of using gravity and the body's own weight to provide resistance, as calisthenics do, free weight training, or weight lifting, uses different pieces of minimal equipment to supply resistance. That equipment includes barbells, dumbbells, weight plates, locking collars, and a bench. Additional equipment is required for some exercises.

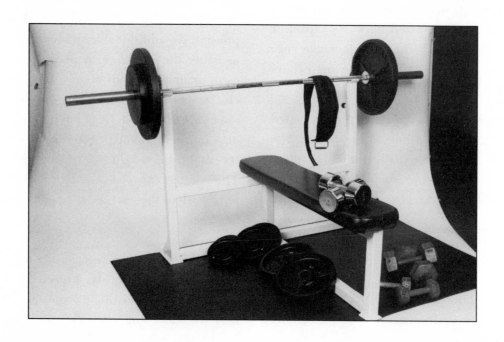

Equipment is available at most large department stores, sporting goods stores, and many sporting goods resale shops, as well as the occasional garage sale. In addition, all the equipment needed is often found in school gyms, health clubs, and other recreational sites. In purchasing equipment, the following should be considered:

**Weight Bench.** At a minimum, this should be a sturdy, well-constructed bench with a satisfactorily padded bed. There should be solid supports on both sides of one end of the bench to hold a barbell securely. The spacing of the barbell supports and width of the bench should be sufficient to allow the arms and elbows to move freely up and down. An advantage is a bench that has the attachment to allow for leg curls and extensions and an adjustable back that can be angled.

**Barbells.** A single, straight barbell is sufficient for most exercises. Most barbells available today use removable weight plates so that the weight can be adjusted to the individual or exercise. Be sure to choose a bar that has solid locking collars on each end to hold the weights firmly.

**Dumbbells.** Dumbbells come as both fixed-weight, one-piece, items or as adjustable models that use the same removable weight plates as the barbell. A single pair of short dumbbell bars are sufficient for most people. As with the barbell, make sure the dumbbell bars have sufficient locking collars to secure all of their weight plates.

**Weights.** These come most often as plastic-coated or plain iron disks with a hole in the center. The plastic-coated disks are usually the cheapest to purchase and come in sizes of $2^1/_2$, 5, and 10 pounds. Plastic plates are also available in 15 and 20 pounds, but these are more difficult to locate. The plastic on the plates wears somewhat with use but also prevents the weights from marring most floors.

The iron plates are the more professional model and come in a wider range of sizes including

45 pounds but are more expensive and represent a major investment. Have enough weight to duplicate the individual's body weight, less the weight of the bar. Four of the $2^1/_2$ pound plates, six of the 5-pound, and the balance in 10-pound and some heavier plates are enough for most uses.

**Weight belt.** This is also known as a kidney belt in some circles. The belt is made up from a variety of materials; leather, nylon, and various cloths have all been used. The belt is very wide in the back and is intended to be worn around the waist, but covers most of the lower back. The purpose of the belt is to help maintain the straightness of the lower back during a movement. Keeping the lower back straight helps minimize stress and the possibility of injury. Purchase a quality belt that fits well, securing around the waist at about the middle of the belt's adjustment to allow for growth or reduction.

## SAFETY

Though no exercise routine should be done alone, the use of free weights more than any other form of exercise requires an additional person to be present. An additional individual acts as a spotter, assisting the exerciser in preparing for a movement or in getting out of one. More than anything else, a spotter acts as a safety feature. If the exerciser gets in trouble from having too much weight on a bar or becoming tired during a set, the spotter can lift the weight before any injury can occur. The spotter can also assist in slightly lifting the weight when the exerciser is pushing on that last, hard rep.

*Note.* More than one experienced weight lifter has been killed or seriously injured by working out with free weights without a spotter. The situation may seem amusing when the weight from a bench press settles down on an exerciser's chest and the individual is pinned. The amusement stops when the ribs break or the bar slips to the individual's neck and presses down.

Some of the exercises described below require the use of some form of weight machine. These can be relatively simple machines with a pivoting or moving section to which you add weight, in the form of weight plates, or complicated devices that utilize weight stacks, springs, elastic, or hydraulics to supply resistance. The inherent safety of most weight machines often eliminates any need for a spotter. Exercises performed on machines can be very specific as to which muscles or groups of muscles they work.

On the negative side, weight machines are very expensive to purchase and maintain so are normally out of the range of most people's budget. Movements on the machines are limited, primarily for safety, and so they are much less dynamic than free weight exercises. Access to weight machines can often be found through gyms or health clubs, usually requiring the purchase of a membership. Many schools, colleges, and universities have machine-equipped weight rooms available to students, and occasionally others, free or at a nominal fee.

When using a new model of weight machine, while on a trip or at a new facility, begin the exercise routine at a lower weight. Machines of different makes may apply resistance to the movement differently. Starting out with a lower weight prevents stressing the muscles excessively before getting the "feel" for a new machine.

The dynamic motion of an exercise, that is the free play of the body against the resistance, varies with the type of weight resistance you are using. This leads to a problem in determining which kind of weight resistance to use. Some individuals swear totally by using weight machines, which have their benefits and drawbacks. And others far prefer the simpler free weights of barbells and dumbbells. Which form of weight resistance is best is determined partially by the kind of exercise being performed, the results desired, and the taste of the individual.

Dumbbells allow the greatest flexibility of motion when using free weights. The arms remain separate in their efforts and do not support each other in moving the load. This separate action allows the weaker arm to do a full amount of the work in a movement, maintaining a symmetry of development between the muscle groups on both sides of the body. This is especially important when recovering from an injury or some other cause that has made one side noticeably weaker than the other. Using the dumbbells weight allows a greater number of reps to be performed by the weaker side or an increase or decrease in the weight used on one side as needed.

Barbells allow a certain flexibility of motion during an exercise, less than that of dumbbells, while permitting the arms to support each other in working against the resistance. The movement of the barbell forces the arms to work together in keeping the bar balanced and level while allowing the stronger arm to take up a slightly greater share of the load. This action enables the arms to move a greater weight together than they could separately. If an individual can bench-press two 40-pound dumbbells, for the same numbers of sets and reps, that same individual could work a 100-pound-plus barbell.

Machines offer the least amount of free motion in an exercise as they concentrate their resistance against a specific muscle group. This allows for the greatest amount of work for a given weight to be concentrated on an area for development. The movement of resistance in a machine is also smoother and much safer in general than the same movement done with free weights. Part of this safety comes from being able to fully support or brace those portions of the body that are not directly involved with the exercise. This benefit particularly protects the lower back from excessive strain. Additional safety comes from the movement limiters built into a machine that normally prevent a weight from being able to drop on or excessively bear against the body.

Where applicable, the free weight exercises listed here show all of the weight resistance options, given in order of importance.

Start doing an exercise at a weight that allows you to complete 3 sets of 12 repetitions each using the correct technique and control. When you are able to complete 3 sets of 15 to 20 reps each of an exercise, increase the weight until you are just able to complete 3 sets of 12 reps each and continue.

## FREE WEIGHT EXERCISES

❏

BENCH PRESS
OVERHEAD (MILITARY) PRESS
UPRIGHT ROW
ARM (BARBELL) CURL
OVERHEAD (BENCH) TRICEPS
EXTENSION
REVERSE CURLS
LEG PRESS
LEG CURLS (KNEE FLEXIONS)
LEG (KNEE) EXTENSIONS
CALF (HEEL) RAISES

❏

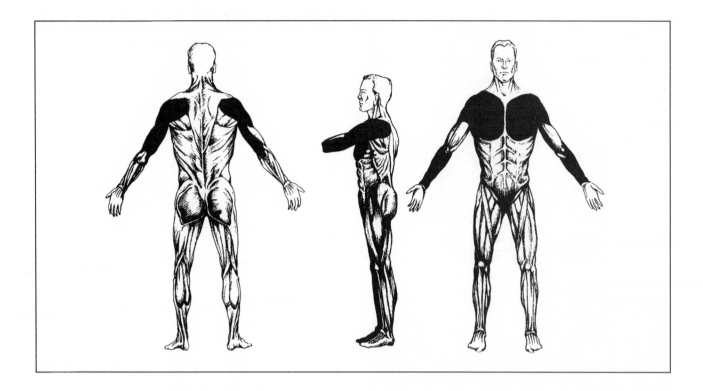

## BENCH PRESS

**Muscle groups.** Upper body, shoulders, and arms, especially the pectoralis major, triceps, deltoids, and the flexor muscles of the forearm.

The bench press is the most commonly done weight lifting exercise and is the primary upper-body movement. It builds up the major muscles used in lifting or pushing with the arms. This development is also visible in the definition of the muscles of the chest.

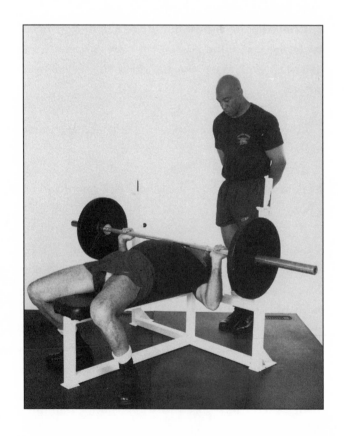

### Technique

1. Lie face-up flat on the bench, placing the legs bent and to either side of the bench, or in whatever position is most comfortable. With the arms extending upward, grasp the barbell with the hands in a pronated (palms out) grip, spaced slightly greater than shoulder-width apart. Lower the bar to the chest slowly and under control. The bar should be centered at the middle of the chest, roughly the nipple area in men.

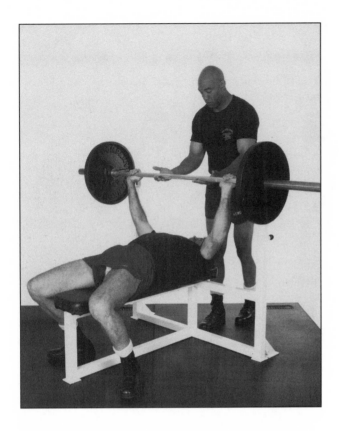

2. From the down position, press the bar straight up to the maximum reach of the arms. Exhale on the push and move the bar in a single, smooth motion.

3. Lower the bar in a slow, controlled motion back to the chest.

**Repetition.** The above completes one repetition of a bench press.

**Advantages.** This is a very basic weight lifting movement and a number of other exercises have developed from it. The bench press maintains its value throughout the extent of a workout program.

**Disadvantages.** This exercise requires a bench. If a bench with weight supports is not available, a plain bench can be used with the spotter handing the exerciser the barbell.

**Recommendations.** Dumbbell presses from a flat or slightly up-angled bench are best as they give the greatest stretch to the pectoral muscle group. The stretch is accomplished in the down position with the dumbbells being lowered past the sides of the chest. The weights may be held parallel to the shoulders or rotated so that they lie in line with the body. Rotate the weights so that they are parallel with the shoulders when in the fully up position.

The barbell is the second best source of weight resistance in the bench press. Because the body can work a greater amount of weight with a barbell than separate dumbbells, and barbells are normally adjustable to a much heavier weight, they are the most common source of weight resistance seen in the bench press.

Machine weights are least useful in the bench press as they prevent a full range of motion and balancing of the bar between the arms.

*Note 1.* The bench press is often used as a marker for upper-body strength. Be extremely careful when pressing large weights and do not attempt the exercise without a partner/spotter. Being able to bench-press an individual's own weight is a very good benchmark of progress and can be used as an indication to increase the number of sets or repetitions by a good amount.

*Note 2.* The concentration of resistance to the muscles worked in the bench press can be easily adjusted. For a greater workout to the triceps muscle, use a narrower or closer grip on the bar. Make certain that the grip is not so narrow that the bar cannot be balanced and controlled. To increase the work done by the pectoral muscles, widen the grip on the bar.

**Uses.** With a light bar, less than 50 percent of body weight, the bench press can be used as a buildup for push-ups.

WARNINGS. Do not arch the neck or back while performing a bench press. This motion can injure

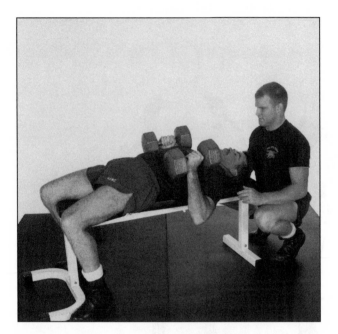

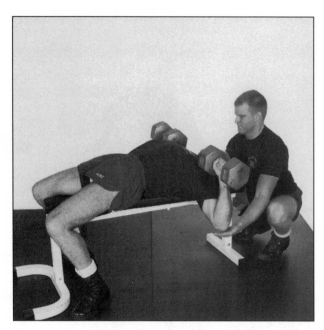

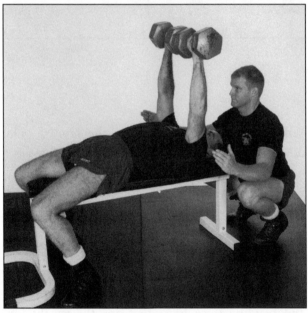

the spine by compressing disks. Do not bounce or drop the weight on the chest to prevent injury to the sternum, ribs, or internal organs. Placing the soles of the feet on the bench is useful for some people in preventing the back from arching. If the weight is too heavy to lift without arching the back, lessen the weight. If there is a chance of dropping the weight toward the chest, lessen the weight or number of repetitions.

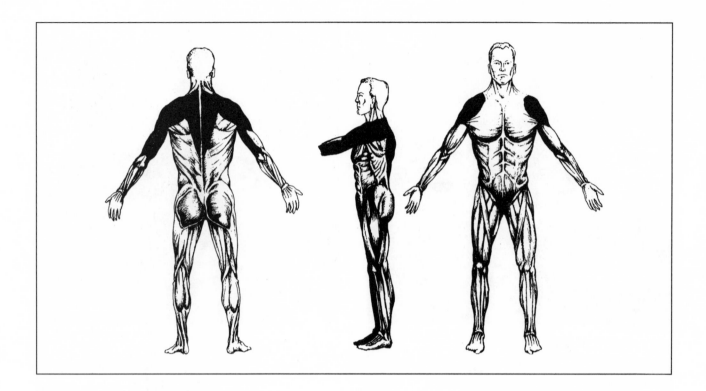

## OVERHEAD (MILITARY) PRESS

**Muscle groups.** Upper arms, shoulders, and upper back, especially the triceps, deltoids, and trapezius.

This press uses movement in a different direction from the bench press to work the muscles of the back as well as the shoulders. The standing version of the movement has benefit for the entire body.

### Technique

1. From an upright, standing position with the feet spaced about shoulder-width apart and the barbell on the ground directly in front of the feet, bend at the knees and squat down behind the bar with the back at a 30-degree angle or less. Keep the back itself straight and bend from the hips. The head is upright and the eyes looking forward.

With the arms straight, place the hands, palm down, on the bar and grasp it firmly.

2. Pull the barbell up past the knees by straightening the legs and hips. Stand upright with the back straight while keeping the knees slightly bent. Use the strength of the legs and hips to raise the weight. Continue the motion smoothly, pushing the hips forward while pulling the shoulders back and bending the elbows to swing the weight forward and up. Swing the barbell up to the chest and rest. The arms are fully bent with the elbows down. The bar rests on the palms of the hand, which faces out from the body, and the wrists are bent so that the weight of the bar bears down on the upright forearm. The barbell should be stationary between the upper chest and chin.

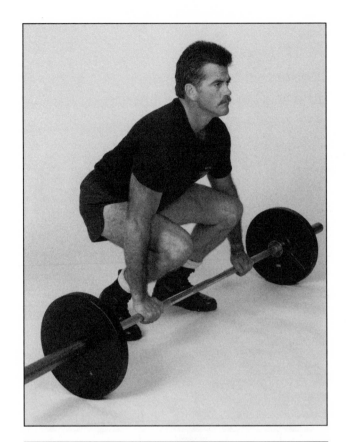

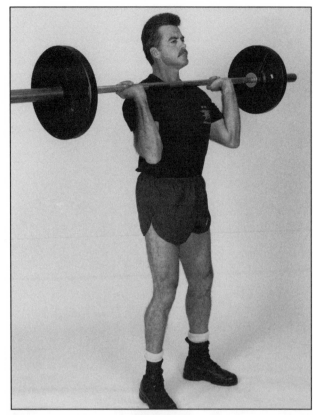

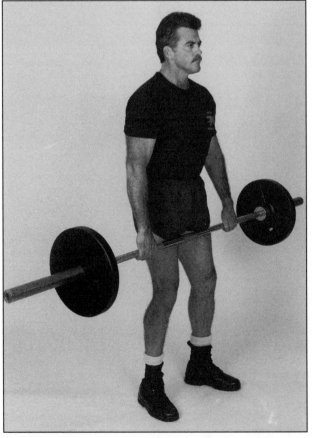

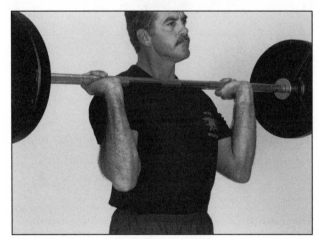

3. Exhale while pushing up with the arms, driving the bar straight up to the maximum reach of the arms. The weight should be kept close to the body and pass near, but not touch, the face.

4. Slowly lower the bar down back to the chest position. Inhale as the bar is coming down.

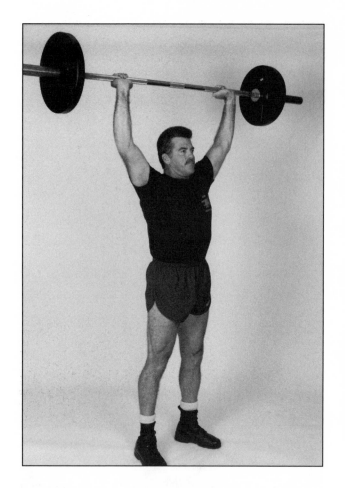

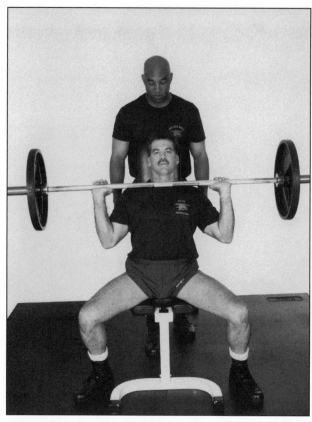

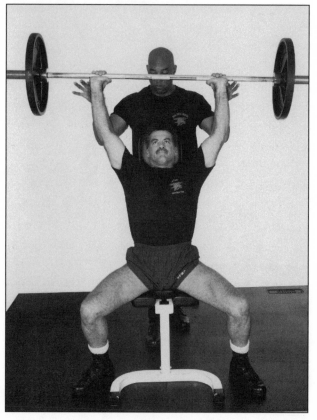

*Note.* After the exercise set is completed, slowly lower the bar back to the ground. Follow the same steps as in the clean (parts 1 and 2) but in reverse order. Do not drop the weight and keep the back straight, bending at the knees, while lowering the weight.

**Repetition.** Parts 3 and 4 of the above complete one repetition of the overhead press. The clean, parts 1 and 2, is not considered when counting repetitions of the exercise.

**Advantages.** This exercise can be done in the standing or seated position with the same effect on the targeted muscle groups.

**Disadvantages.** The back may be easily injured when raising from the crouch while doing the standing version of this movement.

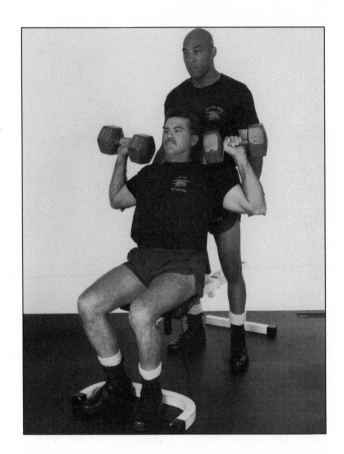 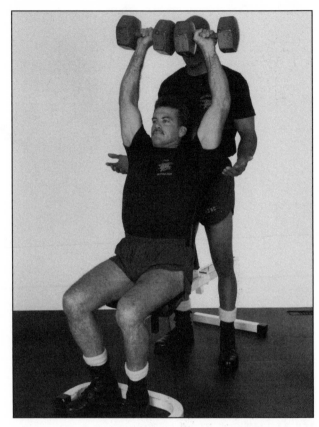

**Recommendations.** Dumbbell overhead presses are the most beneficial as they use the full movement of the shoulders and give the greater stretch to the down movement. The weights may be held in line with the shoulders or rotated so that the palms · face in to the body and the weights are square to the shoulders. Rotate the weights while extending so that they are in line with the shoulders when in the fully up position.

The barbell is the second best source of weight resistance in the overhead press. The bar cannot be brought in line with the shoulders when in the fully down position.

Machine weights are least useful in the over- head press as they limit the range of motion and eliminate balancing of the weight between the arms.

WARNINGS. An improperly done clean can lead to permanent injury. When first doing the clean, guidance and direction should be sought from an experienced, knowledgeable coach or trainer. A weight belt should be worn with this, and with all overhead, unsupported lifts. When standing in the clean, do not arch the back to the rear excessively as it may injure the lower back. Make certain there is sufficient overhead clearance before attempting the standing overhead press.

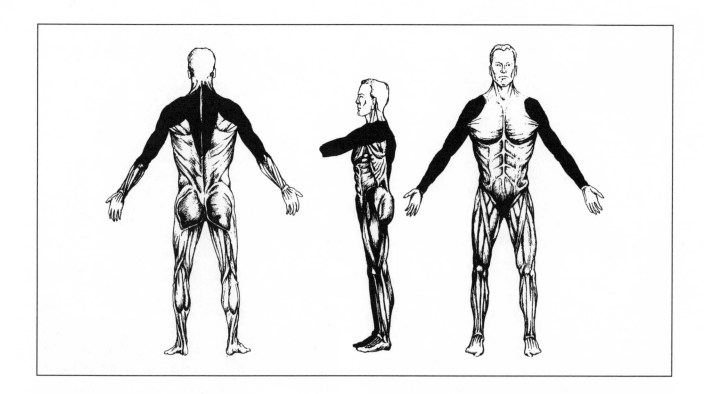

## UPRIGHT ROW

**Muscle groups.** Forearms, upper arms, shoulders, and upper back including the forearm flexors, biceps, triceps, deltoids, rhomboids, and trapezius.

This is considered one of the best upper-body exercises and is one of the most difficult. Heavy stress is placed on the shoulders, upper arms, and back due to the mechanical disadvantage the muscles have in the movement.

### Technique

1. From an upright, standing position with the feet spaced shoulder-width apart or closer, bend at the knees and squat down with the back at a 30-degree angle or less. Keep the back itself straight and bend from the hips. The bar is on the ground directly in front of the feet. The head is held upright throughout the movement and the eyes remain looking forward. With the arms straight, place the hands in the middle of the bar, spaced

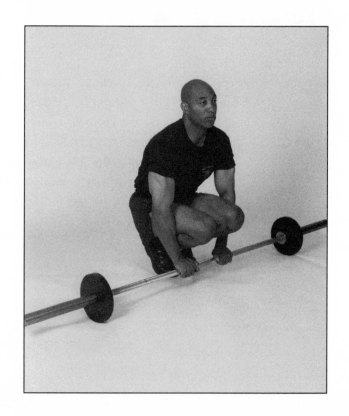

about 4 inches apart with the palms down, and grasp it firmly.

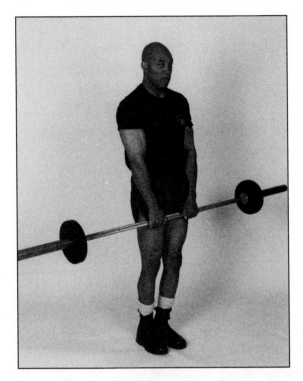

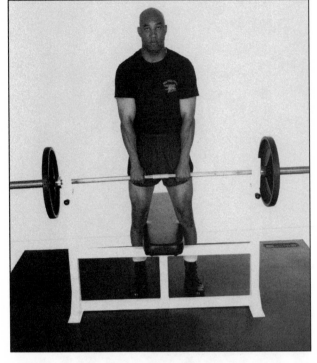

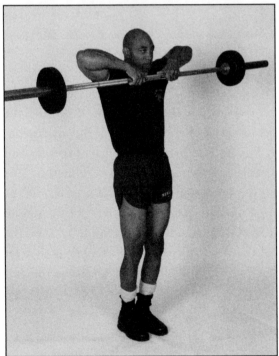

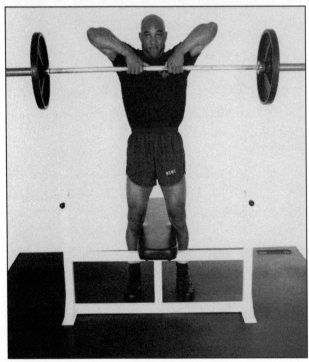

2. Pull the barbell up past the knees to the thighs by straightening the legs and hips. Stand upright with the back straight while keeping the knees slightly bent.

3. Smoothly pull the bar up to stop underneath the chin. Exhale during the lift and lift the bar straight up. The elbows remain higher than the hands throughout the movement. Pause with the bar held up underneath the chin.

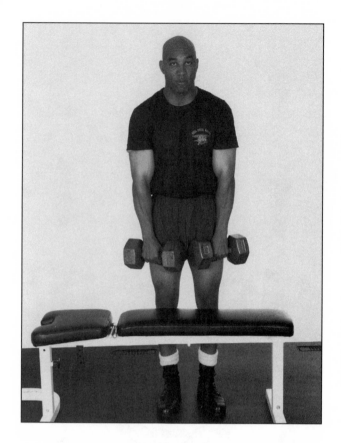
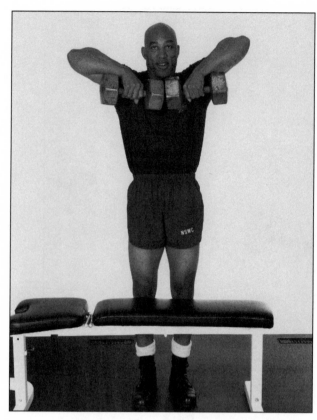

4. Slowly lower the bar back to the hanging position in front of the thighs. Inhale as the bar is lowered into position.

5. To lower the bar down to the floor, bend at the knees and hips, keeping the back straight, until the bar reaches the ground.

**Repetition.** Steps 3 and 4 of the above complete one full repetition of the upright row. Lifting up and putting the bar down to the floor from the standing position are only done once per set.

**Advantages.** Works almost the entire upper body with some benefit to the chest, legs, and lower back.

**Disadvantages.** This is a very difficult exercise to complete. Begin with a very light bar and work the weight up carefully and in small increments.

**Recommendations.** Dumbbells provide the best source of weight for this exercise as they offer the greatest range of motion and work the arms separately. The barbell limits the range of motion and is more difficult to handle in the movement.

One of the better forms of this exercise is the seated row performed at a machine. In the seated row, the weight handle is drawn fully into the lower abdomen on the draw. The handle is then let out slowly to the full stretch of the arms to complete the movement.

WARNINGS. A weight belt support is suggested. Keep the back straight during all parts of the movement to prevent excess stress to the lower back.

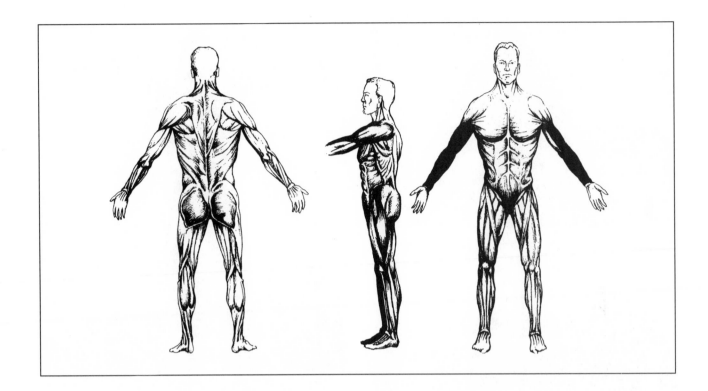

## ARM (BARBELL) CURL

**Muscle groups.** Upper and lower arms, especially the biceps and forearm flexors.

This movement strongly works the upper arms, developing the pulling-action muscles. Use of a free weight helps develop the arms evenly and build balance.

### Technique

1. From a standing position, bend and "clean" the bar up with an undergrip (palms facing away from the body). Keep the elbows tucked in to the sides of the body and the forearms facing forward.

2. Lift (curl) the bar up from in front of the thighs to touch the upper chest, just below the collarbone. Lift the bar in a semicircle by flexing and bending at the elbows and keeping the upper arms still at the sides of the chest. Exhale on the upward motion and pause when the bar reaches the chest. Keep the back straight and upright during the movement. If necessary, the movement can be done with the back up against a wall for additional support.

*Note 1.* At the beginning of the upward movement of the bar, bending or cocking the wrists up and in will add to the workout for the forearms.

*Note 2.* "Cramp" or flex the biceps when the bar is at the top of its movement. Leverage makes the weight of the bar at its least effective at the top of the movement and cramping or "making a muscle" gives added benefit to the biceps.

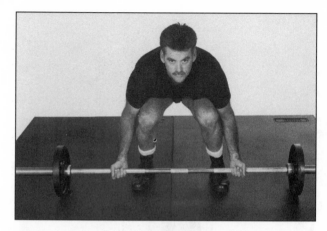

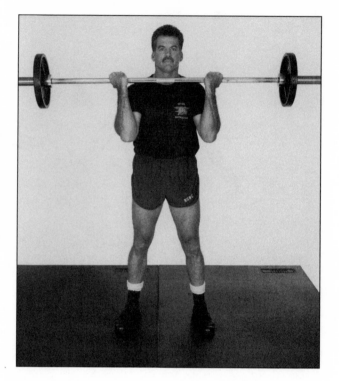

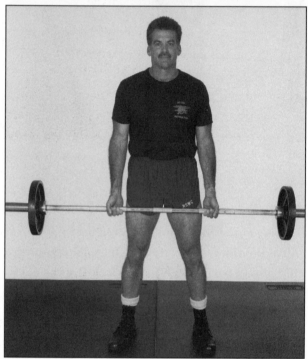

3. Slowly lower the bar in a semicircular motion by straightening the arms, keeping the upper arms in place and moving the forearms. Inhale on the downward motion.

4. Lower the bar from the cleaned position by bending at the knees and hips.

**Repetition.** Steps 2 and 3 of the above complete one repetition of the barbell curl. Cleaning the bar up and down is only done once per set.

**Advantages.** This is a popular exercise that directly benefits the upper arms and overall arm strength.

**Disadvantages.** There is very little resistance to the muscles in the last third of the movement due to the leverage of the arm. It is very easy to swing the weight to assist in the lift or to lift with the shoulders rather than just with the biceps by pivoting the forearm at the elbow.

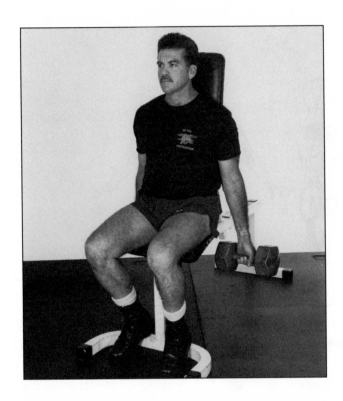

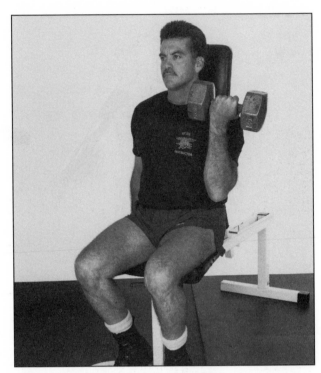

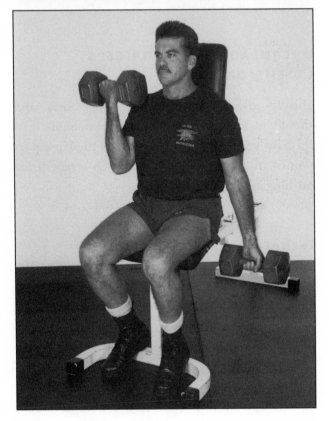

**Recommendations.** Dumbbell curls are the best form of this exercise as they prevent favoring one arm over the other and increase the range of motion for the movement. Dumbbell curls may also be done alternating the up motion between the arms. At the top of the up motion, flex in with the biceps, "peaking" the muscle for the maximum workout.

Barbells and machine (cable) forms of this exercise are roughly the same in terms of benefits with some slight advantage in motion going to the barbell. The barbell and cable handle cannot be drawn in past the chest to assist in peaking the biceps.

WARNINGS. Do not bend the back at any time when doing this movement; injury to the lower back may result. Do not move the hips forward to help swing up the bar. Use a weight belt for additional support when doing this exercise, especially with heavier weights. If the forearms become sore after a few weeks, try to use a specially shaped curl bar.

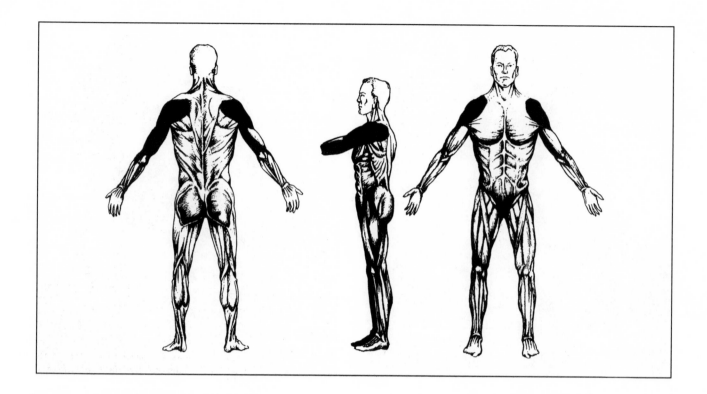

## OVERHEAD (BENCH) TRICEPS EXTENSION

**Muscle groups.** Back of the upper arms and shoulders, primarily the triceps and deltoids.

This exercise specifically works the back portion of the upper arm. It builds up strength for pushing and throwing motions.

### Technique

1. Pick up a light barbell with the hands spaced 6 to 12 inches apart in a palm-down grip. Lie back on a plain, straight bench so that the head hangs over the end of the bench. Place the feet and legs in any comfortable, stable position. Starting with the barbell resting on the chest, straighten the arms to their fully extended position, raising the bar straight up from the chest. The arms should be straight with the forearms and palms of the hands facing toward the feet.

2. Slowly lower the arms toward the head, so that the bar will pass the top of the head without contacting it. Bend the arms at the elbows while moving the bar. End the movement when the bar is hanging down below the head with the elbows bent 90 degrees and the upper arms next to the head and parallel to the bench, or as close to this position as it can be lowered. Inhale on the downward movement. Pause at the end of the movement.

3. Exhale slowly while lifting the bar back up to the starting position by straightening the arms. Simultaneously move the elbows in a semicircular motion, pivoting at the shoulder, while straightening the arms.

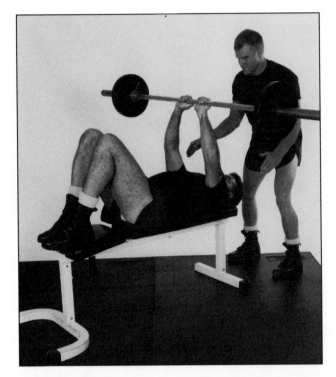

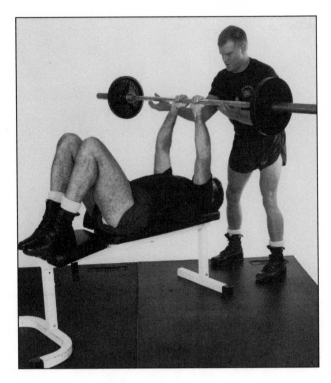

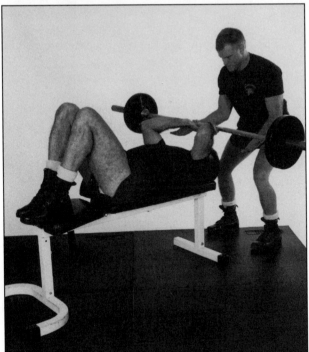

**Repetition.** Steps 2 and 3 of the above complete one bench triceps extension.

**Advantages.** This exercise isolates the triceps muscle for specific attention.

**Disadvantages.** It is a difficult exercise. Use of a specially shaped curl bar can minimize the stress on the forearms.

**Recommendations.** The dumbbell form of this exercise is the best as it gives the best range of motion and workout to the shoulder and triceps. The movement is best done lying on a flat bench, holding the barbells in line with the body with the palms facing in. Extend the weights up from the chest and, bending the arms at the elbows, move them back toward the shoulders. When the elbows reach a 90-degree angle, rotate the upper arms back, moving the weight back over the shoulders. Smoothly move the weight back up, out, and down, reversing the motions of the exercise, to complete the repetition.

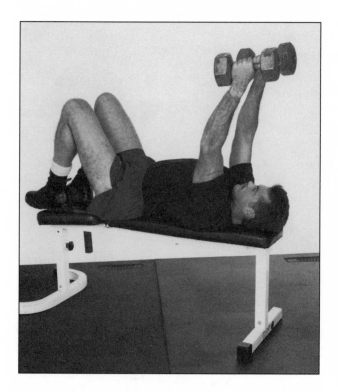

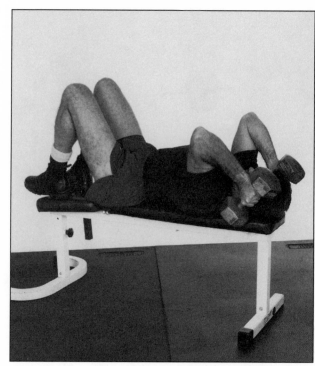

The machine form of this exercise is next in importance, done with a rope handle and pulled down from a cable rig. While in an upright posture, keep the elbows locked in to the body with the upper arms in line with the torso. Pull the handle down moving the forearms only, spreading the hands slightly as the movement reaches its maximum extension. Slowly move the arms back to the up position to complete the repetition.

The barbell form of the triceps extension is the most difficult version of the movement.

WARNINGS. Use minimum weight when beginning this exercise and maintain positive control against the resistance at all times. Loss of control of the barbell particularly can result in a serious injury to the head.

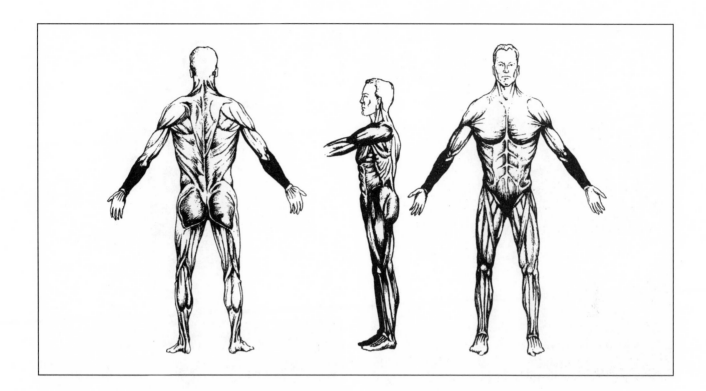

## REVERSE CURLS

**Muscle groups.** Forearms, particularly the forearm flexors and extensors.

This exercise isolates and develops the muscles of the forearm and wrist. These muscles add to grip strength. The movement can be done to aid one group of muscles at a time, either the extensors on the outside or the flexors on the inside of the forearm.

## Technique

1. The exercise can be conducted in a standing or sitting position. Start with a pronated (palm down) grip on either the dumbbell or barbell weight. If using a barbell, space the hands shoulder-width apart. In the standing position, hold the upper arms straight down along the chest, with the elbows bent out to lower the weight to in front of the thighs.

2. Lift the weight by curling the wrist back and raising the upper arms to their maximum extent.

3. Slowly lower the weight down to the starting position, uncurling the wrist during the motion.

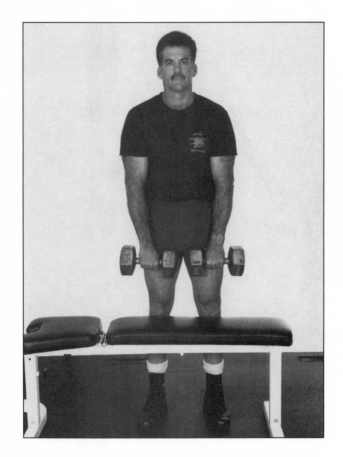

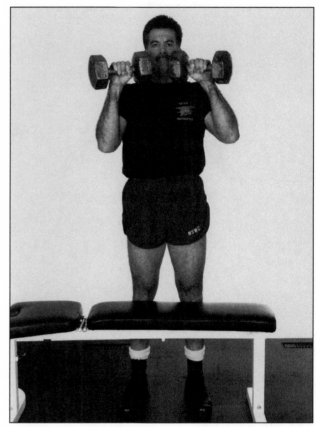

**Repetition.** The above completes one full reverse curl movement.

**Advantages.** This exercise builds up the extensor and flexor muscles specifically. The curl of the wrist while moving the weight isolates the forearm flexor muscles. The exercise can use either barbells, separate dumbbells, or a machine.

**Disadvantages.** This is a difficult and advanced exercise and requires some forearm strength before beginning. Standard upper-body free weight exercises will build up the forearms over time to the point where the reverse curls can be attempted.

**Recommendations.** The dumbbells form of this exercise has the maximum benefit as it allows the muscles to be peaked at the top of the movement. The machine and then barbell forms follow next in importance as they cannot allow for the peaking action at the top of the movement.

WARNINGS. Begin with a light weight. Discontinue immediately if any forearm pain develops. Do the movement slowly and take care that the weight bar does not slip from the fingers as the hands become tired.

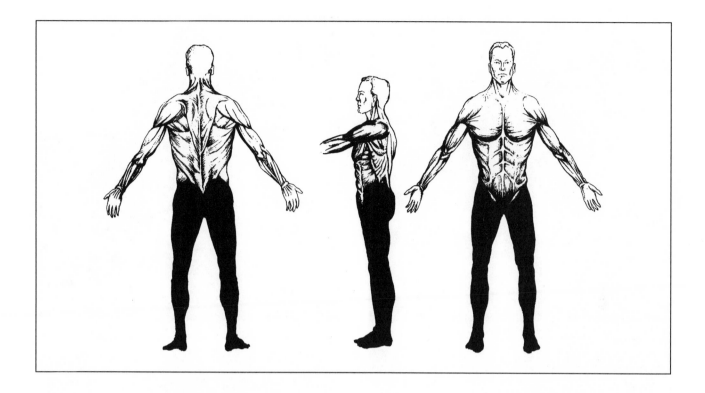

## LEG PRESS

**Muscle groups.** The upper and lower legs and the buttocks, particularly the quadriceps femoris, hamstrings, gastrocnemius, soleus, and plantaris muscles as well as the gluteus maximus.

This is a machine-based exercise performed on any one of a number of leg-press machines. The movement builds up the strength of the entire leg.

### Technique

1. Adjust the machine so that the body can enter a firm, supported position and the legs will be bent at a 90-degree angle prior to any movement taking place. Set the weight of the machine as needed. Sit or lie in the machine as required, placing the feet on the pressure plate. Grasp any handgrips pro-

vided for safety and support. Unlock the machine's moving parts if necessary.

2. Exhale slowly and push with the balls of the feet, keeping the soles of the feet in contact with the pressure plate. Push the plate until the legs are fully extended and pause. Keep the knees slightly bent when the legs are extended.

3. Retract the legs slowly, maintaining control of the weight. Inhale on the negative movement. Return the pressure plate or weight stack to their original position.

*Note.* After the set is over, replace or reset any safety or movement locks on the machine.

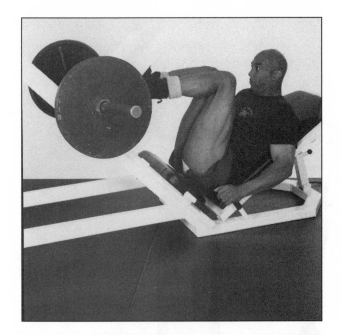

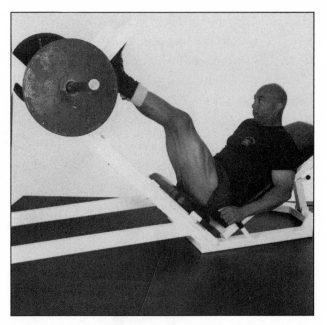

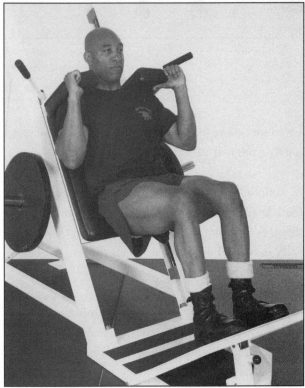

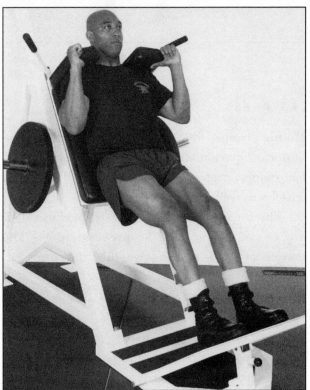

**Repetition.** Steps 2 and 3 complete one repetition of a leg press.

**Advantages.** This is a much safer and more convenient movement than the squat, which works the same muscles.

**Disadvantages.** This exercise requires access to a leg-press machine.

**Recommendations.** The leg-press machine that allows you to lie back and push up or out with the legs is the preferred apparatus. Going deeper than a 90-degree bend at the knees increases the benefit to the buttocks and hamstrings while increasing the stress on the lower back.

A standing, or "hack squat," leg-press machine can put severe stress on the lower back and knees. In this, do not lower the body any deeper than halfway, knees at 90 degrees, to prevent injury.

WARNINGS. Considerable stress can be put on the lower back in this exercise. Do not use too heavy a weight, and start conservatively. Wear a weight belt if available. If any discomfort is felt in the back, stop the exercise immediately and use a lighter weight during the next workout session. Do not lock the knees when the legs are in the fully extended position.

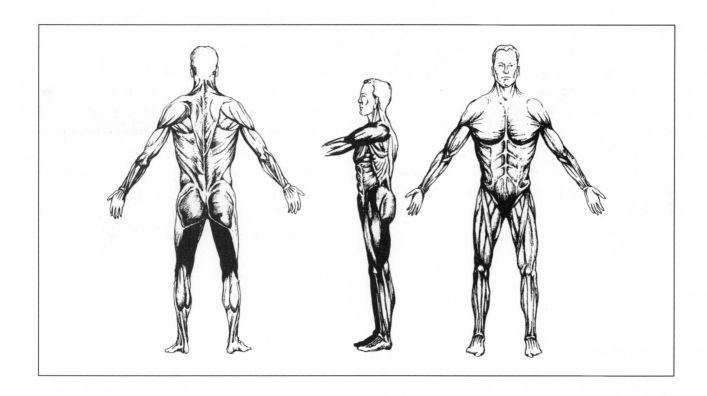

## LEG CURLS (KNEE FLEXIONS)

**Muscle groups.** Back of the thighs, concentrating on the hamstrings and specifically the biceps femoris.

This is a machine exercise that works the muscles at the upper rear of the leg. These muscles perform a pull action with the leg such as would be done during a downstroke while swimming with fins.

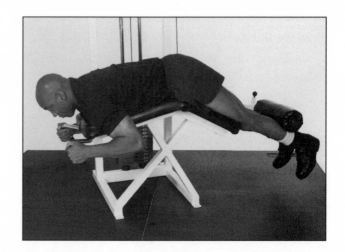

### Technique

1. Adjust the bed, seat, or pressure pad of the machine so that the pressure of the exercise will be transmitted from the back of the ankles or lower calves. Set the weight of the machine as needed. Lie or sit on the support as required with the legs in position. Hold any handgrips available for support.

2. Exhale slowly and flex the knees, bringing the lower legs back toward the buttocks. Close the flex as much as possible, either contacting the buttocks or reaching the limit of the machine. Pause at the point of maximum knee flexion.

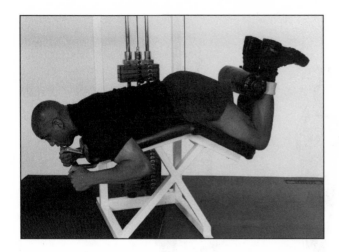

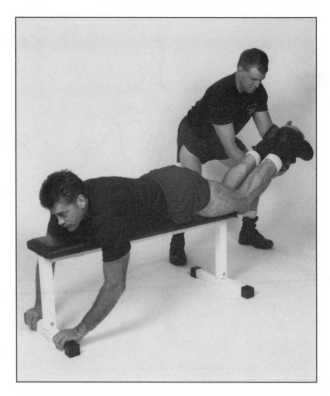

3. Inhale while returning the leg to the extended position slowly in a smooth, controlled manner.

*Note.* If a leg-curl machine is not available, a reasonable workout can be obtained with a dumbbell. Lie down on a flat bench and hold the dumbbell between the feet. Perform the leg curl as above in steps 2 and 3, being careful to hold the dumbbell securely throughout the movement.

**Repetition.** Steps 2 and 3 of the above complete one repetition of the leg curl.

**Advantages.** This exercise concentrates action on the back of the thigh in the safest and easiest movement. The exercise can be done with a simple attachment on some weight benches.

**Disadvantages.** Requires access to a leg-curl machine or attachment.

WARNINGS. Take extreme care if using the dumbbell option that the weight is securely held.

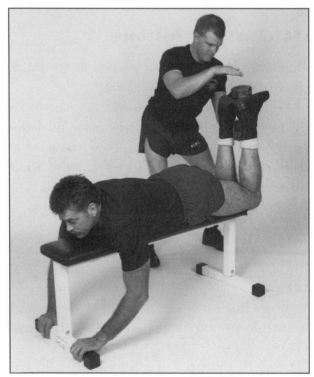

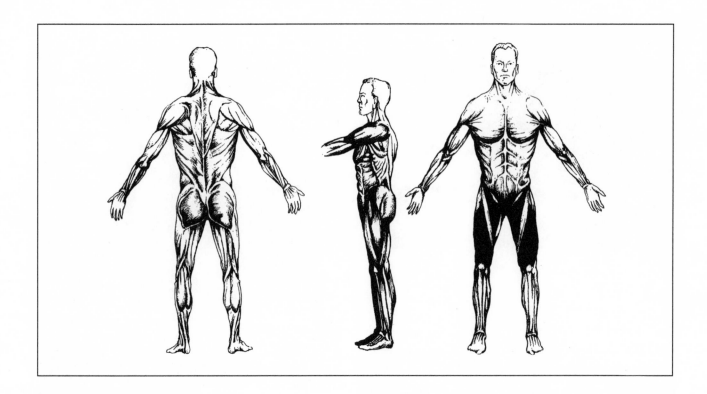

## LEG (KNEE) EXTENSIONS

**Muscle groups.** The front portion of the thigh, specifically the quadriceps femoris.

This machine exercise works the muscles at the front of the leg. The muscles move the lower leg forward in a push stroke. Slow extension of these muscles are used in flutter kicks or while swimming with fins on the forward stroke. The muscles also work explosively such as in the kicking action of the lower leg.

## Technique

1. Adjust the seat or pressure pad of the machine so that the pressure of the exercise will be trans-

mitted from the front of the shin, just above the ankles. Set the weight of the machine as needed. Sit on the support as required, bending the legs to get into position. Grasp any handgrips available for stability.

2. While exhaling slowly, extend the knees until the legs are straight. Pause and hold the position at maximum extension.

3. Inhale while slowly returning the legs to the bent position. Move the weight back into place slowly and smoothly.

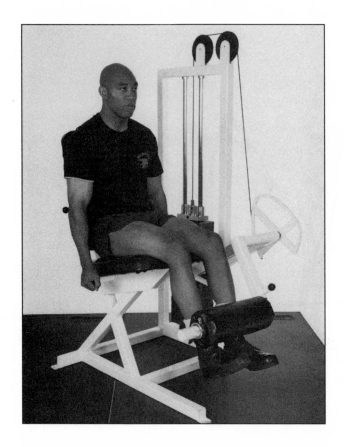 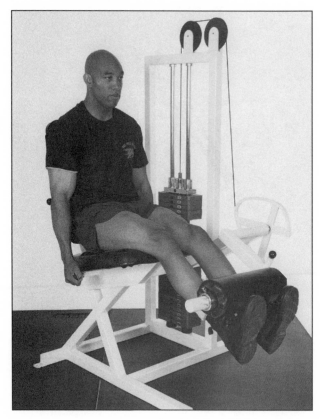

**Repetition.** Steps 2 and 3 of the above complete one repetition of a leg extension.

**Advantages.** This exercise builds up the upper front of the leg with minimum stress. It also increases strength in the muscles that support the kneecap, eliminating pain from some injuries.

**Disadvantages.** The exercise requires a machine. The movement can cause kneecap pain in some individuals.

WARNINGS. This exercise causes kneecap pain in some individuals. Stop exercising immediately if any sharp discomfort is felt in the knees during the movement. Report the pain to a physician.

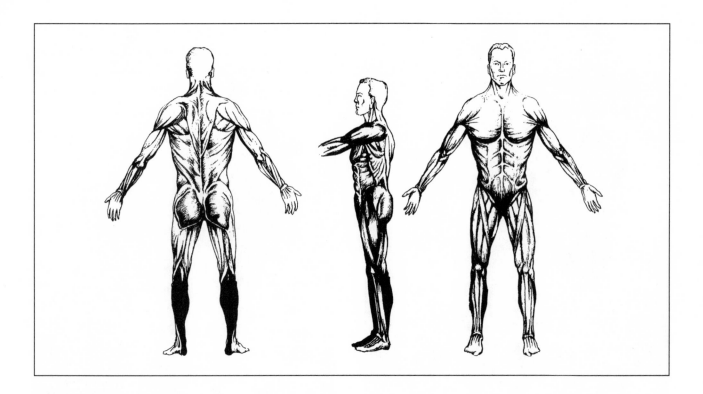

## CALF (HEEL) RAISES

**Muscle groups.** Back of the lower leg, especially the gastrocnemius, soleus, and plantaris muscles.

    This exercise builds up the strong muscles at the back of the lower leg. The calf muscles require a heavy resistance for their size but only a movement of a few inches at most in the heel. This particular movement is a low-impact, weight-intensified version of the calisthenic exercise that concentrates its action almost fully on the targeted muscles.

### Technique

1. To begin, hold a light barbell securely in front of the shoulders, palm up. The barbell may also be held in a comfortable grip with the arms extended down in front of the body and the bar in front of the waist. Alternatively, a set of dumbbells may be used, one in each hand, with the arms hanging down to the sides. Stand on the edge of a stair or block of wood a few inches thick, with the heels out over the edge of the support. Slowly lower the

heels as much as possible while still being able to maintain balance.

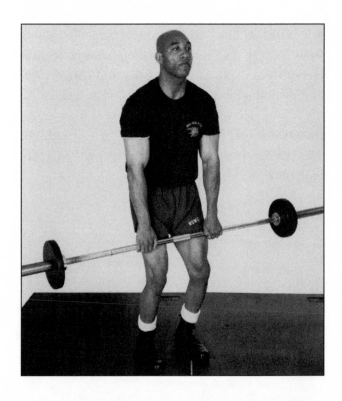

fully extended, press the pressure plate further by pushing with the balls of the feet. Extending and retracting the front of the foot is the same as one repetition of a calf raise. The calf raises can be added at the end of a leg-press routine.

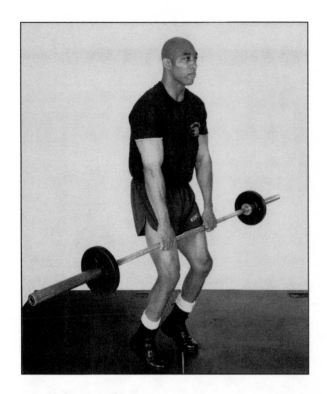

2. Raise the body slowly up on the balls of the feet and toes to the maximum extension of the foot. Keep the body in an upright posture. Contract and peak the calf muscles at the top of the movement and pause.

3. Slowly lower the heels in a smooth movement.

**Repetition.** Steps 2 and 3 of the above complete one full repetition of the calf raise.

**Advantages.** This exercise can be done with free weights or a machine. Beginning exercises may be done with no weight at all.

**Disadvantages.** It is difficult to maintain balance while performing the movement on a stair or block. Use one hand against a solid brace where possible while maintaining a stable grip on the barbell. A partner may also help maintain balance while the exercise is being learned.

*Note.* This exercise can also be performed on some leg-press machines. In the leg press, with the legs

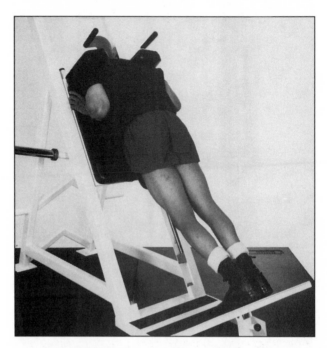

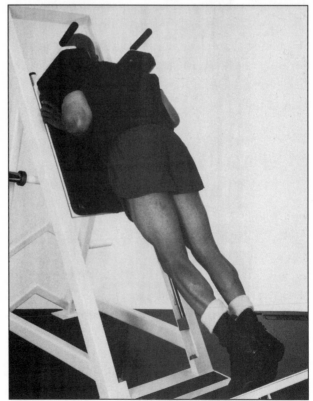

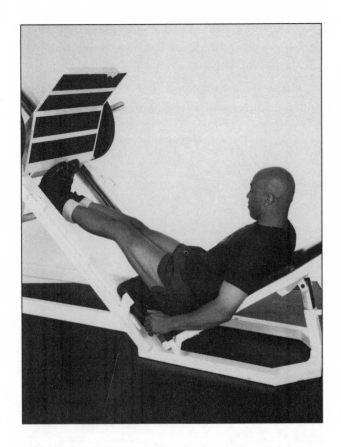
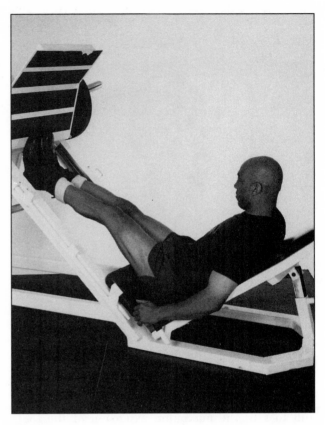

**Recommendations.** The leg-press-machine version of this exercise is the most preferred form as it isolates the calves most efficiently. When performing the exercise on the machine, lower the heels fully in the movement to work the front portion of the calves.

WARNINGS. Take care if placing the barbell across the shoulders that it does not strike and injure the back of the neck or head.

# RUNNING

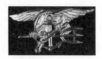

By any name, it was still the toughest school in the Navy
and probably the whole U.S. military. All of the men at the school,
from the enlisted instructors to the officers, did their best to maintain
the high quality of the graduates of training. These were men
we might have to operate with in combat some day and they were
going to be just as tough and competent as we were.
—SEAL, Class 17

ONE OF THE most popular cardiovascular workouts is to go on a run. Distance or timed runs work a majority of the muscles of the body at once. In the Teams, running is an almost constant activity, with distance runs done on a regular basis and many SEALs continuing for additional runs while on their own time. At BUD/S training, running is a constant. Students run to classes, to meals, and to anywhere else their instructors send them. During First Phase it is the unhappy student who is spotted by an instructor walking anywhere in the compound.

For the physical demands put on the lower extremities during BUD/S, running is considered the primary means of preparation. The full weight of the body is raised and lowered constantly during a run or jog. The impact of this movement is absorbed in the bones and joints of the legs. The result of these impacts can be injuries that include stress fractures. For this reason the running workouts listed in Schedule I have no running whatsoever during Week 3. This lack of running allows the bones of the lower legs to adjust to the high levels of stress that they are now under in the workout program. If you are already in a running program, you may continue with the Week 2 running schedule through Week 3.

Running can be at almost any speed from a slow trot to a hard sprint but will be considered for this book as moving at a rate of 11 minutes or less per mile. Running is defined as a form of movement where only one foot is on the ground at any one time and where both feet are in the air at some point on each stride. Walking, on the other hand, is a form of movement where one foot is constantly in contact with the ground. A speed of 13 minutes 45 seconds is considered a good walking pace. Jogging is a slow to moderate run averaging a maximum speed of about 12 minutes per mile. A fast walk can cover ground more quickly than a slow jog. But the primary form of this exercise done in the Teams is the run or sprint.

Proper running form, footwear, and stretching are key to avoiding injury while involved in a running program. Posture while running should be upright, with the back straight and a slight forward lean. This erect posture will be less tiring than one where the shoulders or body is drooping. The head should be kept up and looking forward, focusing the eyes about 10 to 20 yards ahead of the runner. The arms hang loosely and the elbows are bent so that the forearms are held in a relaxed position at the waist. Legs move naturally at the hips with no unnecessary or exaggerated lifting of the feet or knees, and the arms swing naturally in cadence with the legs.

As a very energetic aerobic workout, running develops a lot of body heat. The runner must be properly dressed to prevent overheating while still being protected from chilling at the end of a run. Sweating helps cool the body and prevent overheating. Clothing that blocks the perspiration from evaporating will quickly lead to overheating. Light cotton T-shirts and cotton shorts are the best general uniform for running. Cotton gym pants and sweatshirts offer good protection in cooler weather. Avoid waterproof clothing made of plastic or rubber. In bad weather a nylon windbreaker over a sweatshirt should be sufficient protection without causing overheating.

Probably the most important piece of running equipment is the proper footwear. A quality shoe is necessary for the protection of the feet, while fads and excessive styling add to expense only. Between $50 and $130 can be easily spent on qual-

ity shoes. Follow the advice of a knowledgeable salesperson in making your selection. As the wear on the shoe increases, the protection it offers to the foot decreases. A pair of good running shoes should be replaced every 500 to 700 miles even if no excessive wear is visible. A single quality pair of shoes should last an individual through the 429 to 462 miles of running listed in the workout schedule of this book.

A unique form of running is performed at BUD/S that needs to be practiced by the individual preparing to attend. BUD/S students will regularly run in soft sand while wearing issue combat boots. Part of the running schedule in the workouts should be performed in boots, on sand preferably. The boots may be the modern, nylonsided models, and good, cotton socks should be worn. Sand is one of the most difficult surfaces to run on and beach runs at BUD/S have broken more than one student. Prepare accordingly.

Distance runs are normally practiced as part of a running program. These runs cover over a mile and usually considerably more. The maximum run listed in the workout schedules is eight miles. An individual may run more than this distance but should find himself properly prepared for BUD/S following the listed schedules; there is no need to run the marathon distances recommended in earlier publications. Hard distance runs conducted closely together prevent the body from recovering properly and gaining benefit from the exercise. At worst, excessive running can lead to overtraining with its derogatory effects on the body and mind.

Interval running is an advanced exercise technique that can rapidly build up an individual's speed and overall fitness level. In interval running, a greater than normal pace, though not a sprint, is held while running short distances. Gradually, shorter periods of recovery follow the individual runs. Recovery periods grow shorter while the total number of intervals run increases.

The times for interval runs given in workout

Schedule III are based on the 7-minute-per-mile pace that should be maintained by the end of Schedule II. Rest intervals are best spent slowly walking rather than by standing still.

One change that is making its way through the training program of the Teams is the cutting back on distance runs and increasing slower, weighted runs. In a real-world situation it is even more important to be able to transport a necessary amount of equipment by foot than to just cover the ground quickly. Slower runs conducted while carrying weighted rucksacks address this situation.

A weighted run may be practiced by the individual in place of a regular distance run in Sched-

ule III. A 2- or 4-mile run can be conducted at a minimum 10- to 12-minute-per-mile pace while wearing a rucksack containing sandbags or other yielding weights. The use of a hard weight, such as free weight plates, bricks, or rocks should be avoided due to the threat of possible injury or bruising to the back. A maximum beginning weight should be no more than 20 percent of the individual's body weight. The 20-percent weight should include all clothing, footwear, and equipment carried on the run. Weight runs should not replace distance runs but should instead be used to augment the overall exercise program.

# SWIMMING

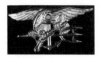

Hell week itself is something that's really just there
as a big blur during training. But that week is the time that
will show whether or not you have the undefinable "it" that will
get you through training and into the Teams. For all of
its physical demands, Hell Week is a test of your mental state
more than anything else. If you don't have it, the "fire in the gut"
as they say today, you just aren't going to make it.

**—SEAL, Class 28**

**I**N NO OTHER Special Operations force does swimming hold as important a place as with the U.S. Navy SEALs. From the very first days of the UDTs in World War II, the water was a safe haven for the men of the Teams. Whether it is used as a concealed means of approaching a target, a way of hiding to prevent discovery, or a means of slipping away unseen after an operation, the men of the Teams have always looked to the water.

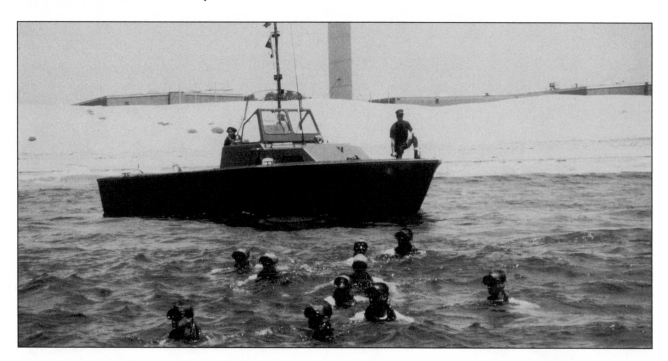

Swimming and working in the water have always been excellent forms of low-impact exercise as well as providing a good overall aerobic workout. While swimming, the body is supported and made buoyant by the displacement of the water. This buoyancy limits the risk of injury to the joints or muscles during exercise. This low-impact action allows waterborne exercises to be conducted by injured or recovering individuals.

Most water work done in the Teams involves straightforward swimming. Freestyle swimming is normally conducted with the crawl stroke. Since it is beyond the scope of this book to teach basic swimming, and the crawl is one of the more basic strokes, it will be assumed that everyone continuing with this program can swim competently. If not, a qualified swimming course is often available from the adult education department of the local schools. Alternatively, the Red Cross swimming course can be taken at a local YMCA or other source.

The most common swim stroke used in the Teams is the sidestroke. The sidestroke is one of the earliest swimming strokes known to the sport and has a reasonably high degree of efficiency for movement in the water. A particular advantage of the sidestroke is that it can be done with a long "glide" portion, allowing it to be used for swimming very long distances with the least expenditure of energy. Additionally, the sidestroke can leave one arm free to tow equipment, or an injured swim buddy. Lastly, the sidestroke can be done with almost no part of the body except the head protruding from the water. This limits what is available to be seen by an observer on shore or aboard ship.

## THE SIDESTROKE

1. The starting position for the sidestroke is lying in the water on the left side. The left arm is extended, palm down, above the head and in line with the body. The right arm is extended back and along the right leg.

2. To begin the stroke, pull the left arm downward, with the arm straight, until it extends straight down from the shoulder. When the left arm extends straight down, flex it in at the elbow and pull it up to the side, turning the palm in toward the face. Then extend the left arm straight back out over the head, back into the starting position.

As the left arm is moving, bring the right arm up by bending it at the elbow. Push the right hand up in front of the chest; then push forward and downward from the face or chin. The right hand pulls back through the water, curving in, until it reaches its starting position by the right leg. The coordination of the movement is as if the left hand was drawing back a handful of water and passing it to the right hand, which continues to push the "handful" back to the rear.

3. The kick with the legs done with the sidestroke is the standard scissors kick performed on the side. To begin the kick, draw the feet up with the right foot ahead of and separated from the left by 12 inches or so. Draw the feet up until the knees are bent to 90 degrees. Straighten the right knee and thrust the foot forward, down, and back in a circular sweep. At the same time, straighten the left leg and thrust the left foot backward, down, and forward in a sweeping kick. The movement of the legs resembles a scissors closing, which is where its name comes from. At the end of the kick, the legs are extended to the rear with the toes pointing backward as the body glides through the water.

The sidestroke can be done with or without swim fins. It is important to get used to swimming with fins on as they are constantly used when swimming in the Teams. Kicking with fins on uses the muscles of the legs in a different manner than other exercises and can quickly cramp up the legs to the point of uselessness when improperly done.

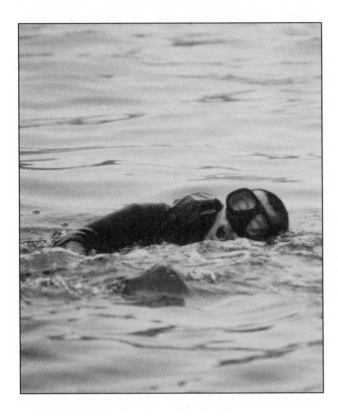

There are two basic types of swim fins on the market, those with a strap that goes around behind the heel to secure the fins to the feet and those with a full pocket that holds the foot. The choice of fins is up to the individual, but the fins preferred in the Teams are an old design known as "duck feet," which have a strap around the heel and a very stiff blade.

The blade of the fin increases the surface area of the foot that pushes against the water. This increased area allows the more powerful leg muscles to propel the body through the water efficiently with little or no assistance from the hands. The action of the fins also greatly increases the stress on the legs and feet. That stress is what can cause cramping so easily when swimming with fins. If you get a cramp while wearing fins, stop and grab the tip of the fin on the foot affected. Pull the tip of the fin up and back and hold it until the cramp eases and then continue.

The individual should choose the size and stiffness of swim fin that gives him the best motion and power without tiring him excessively. Small or soft swim fins should be avoided. A close approximation of the swim fins used in the Teams would be a large, fairly stiff, fin with a securing strap.

When choosing fins, pick a size that allows the wearing of neoprene boots inside the fin. The neoprene boots will protect the foot in the open-strap fins and insulate the foot from cold waters.

A deep, slow, kick is best when wearing fins. Do not try to kick with the same fast, shorter strokes that are done with the bare foot. That kicking style will almost guarantee a bad foot and leg cramp. When fins were first introduced to the UDTs of World War II back in 1944, they were almost immediately abandoned as unfit for use. The experienced swimming instructors then had no experience in swimming with fins on and they badly cramped their legs when using fins. An influx of new personnel from another maritime unit showed the UDT men how to use swim fins and they have been an integral part of the units ever since.

Swimming should be conducted in open waters as much as possible. When a body of open water is not available, a swimming pool is very satisfactory. The open-water swim allows for a straight distance swim workout without the turns needed in a pool. In addition, the usually colder water found in lakes and oceans is good training for a later time at BUD/S. Cold waters abound off Coronado.

Two important swimming skills that are developed at BUD/S are swimming underwater and drownproofing. Drownproofing can only be safely practiced and learned in a pool environment with qualified supervision. THERE IS NO SAFE WAY TO DUPLICATE SOME OF THE DROWN-PROOFING SKILLS PRACTICED AT BUD/S!

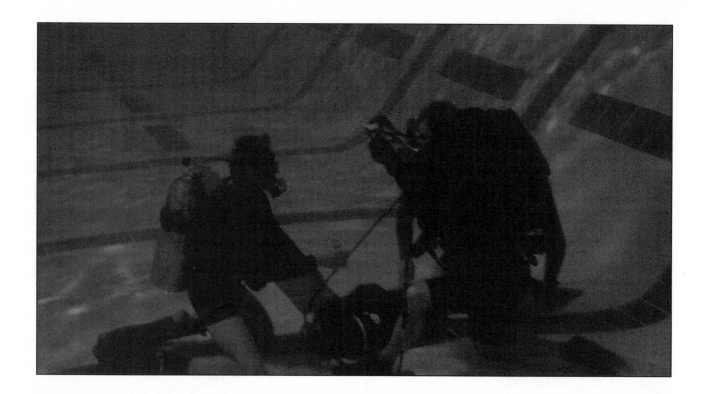

The only practical thing an individual can learn in regards to drownproofing outside of BUD/S is to relax and float in the water. Being able to relax in the water and support yourself with a minimum expenditure of energy is an important skill to have when reporting for BUD/S.

The other major water skill learned at BUD/S is underwater swimming without breathing equipment. That can be practiced simply at the pool by seeing how far you can go underwater on a single breath of air. Just take a deep breath and push off, forcing yourself to swim as far as possible before having to come up for air. Just doing this action regularly will increase the distance you can travel underwater on a single breath. Your kicking and swimming stroke will improve and your body will learn how much it can push itself before having to breathe.

One important note about underwater swimming: A technique for extending your time underwater, known as hyperventilating, has led to the deaths of several swimmers from underwater blackout. Hyperventilating, the forced exhalation

and deep breathing before holding one's breath, is simply too dangerous to be worth its use. DO NOT HYPERVENTILATE WHEN PRACTICING UNDERWATER SWIMMING!

## SCUBA DIVING

Though it is not necessary, it is beneficial to take a basic civilian scuba diving instruction course prior to entering BUD/S. Attending a scuba course will give instruction in basic underwater skills such as clearing a mask, swimming with fins, and general safety procedures. This experience will help an individual recognize and perhaps eliminate any troubles he may find during the civilian training.

There are some disadvantages to taking scuba training before entering BUD/S that should also be considered. All necessary underwater skills will be thoroughly taught at BUD/S in Third Phase. The majority of SEAL underwater work will be conducted with closed-circuit rebreathers that cannot

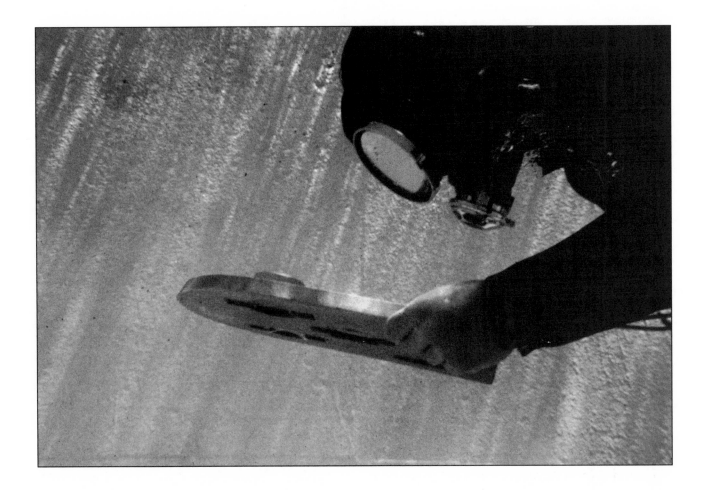

be safely learned in the civilian community. Closed-circuit training is extremely specialized and the use of the system has several inherent dangers. The system uses pure oxygen, which is toxic past certain depths. There is a reason that SEALs earn hazardous duty pay; this is one of them.

In addition, scuba training and the obtaining of equipment can be expensive. Even renting diving gear can quickly add up in cost. The training courses are rarely inexpensive, and only the nationally certified ones should be even considered.

Certified scuba training can be obtained through a number of universities and colleges at relatively low cost. Also, there are usually a large number of civilian dive shops in areas where there are large bodies of water. Most of these shops have a training course available through them or in cooperation with another shop. Only nationally recognized courses of instruction, such as those offered by PADI (Professional Association of Diving Instructors), the YMCA, or the Red Cross, should even be considered.

# WORKOUT SCHEDULES

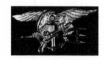

*"Thank God it's Friday" takes on a whole new meaning.*
*It's that Friday, when they secure you from Hell Week,*
*that you know that you have accomplished something that*
*few men will even face, let alone get through.*
**—SEAL, Class 28**

A FIRM RULE IS to always warm up prior to a workout session. No matter what the exercise—calisthenics, weight training, running, or swimming—there will be a greater benefit to the body and a lessened chance of injury if a proper warm-up is done first.

## PHYSICAL TRAINING SCHEDULE I

### WEEK 1

Workout days: Monday, Wednesday, Friday
Warm-up

| PT | Sets | Reps | Exercise |
|----|------|------|----------|
|    | 4    | 15   | Push-ups |
|    | 4    | 20   | Sit-ups  |
|    | 3    | 3    | Pull-ups |

Cool-down

**Swimming (daily if possible)**
Running warm-up
Swim continuously using the sidestroke for 15 minutes.
Running cool-down

**Running**
Running warm-up
Run 2 miles at an 8½-minute-per-mile pace; total, 6 miles per week
Running cool-down

## WEEK 2

Warm-up

| PT | Sets | Reps | Exercise |
|---|---|---|---|
| | 5 | 20 | Push-ups |
| | 5 | 20 | Sit-ups |
| | 3 | 3 | Pull-ups |

Cool-down

### Swimming (daily if possible)

Running warm-up

Swim continuously using the sidestroke for 15 minutes.

Running cool-down

### Running

Running warm-up

Run 2 miles at an 8-minute-per-mile pace; total, 6 miles per week

Running cool-down

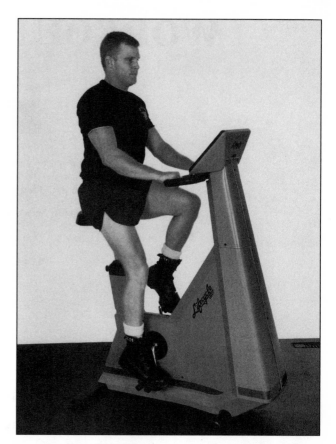

## WEEK 3

Warm-up

| PT | Sets | Reps | Exercise |
|---|---|---|---|
| | 5 | 25 | Push-ups |
| | 5 | 25 | Sit-ups |
| | 3 | 4 | Pull-ups |

Cool-down

### Swimming (daily if possible)

Running warm-up

Swim continuously using the sidestroke for 10 minutes without fins.

Swim continuously using the sidestroke for 10 minutes with fins.

### Running

No running at all during Week 3; there is a very high risk of stress injuries to the legs. Bicycle or use a stationary bicycle/stair climber for 15 minutes in place of running. Do the running warm-up prior to bicycling or other run replacement.

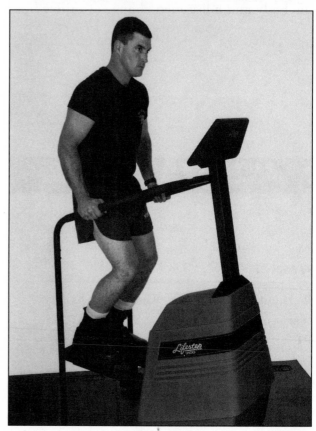

## WEEK 4

Warm-up

| PT | Sets | Reps | Exercise |
|---|---|---|---|
| | 5 | 25 | Push-ups |
| | 5 | 25 | Sit-ups |
| | 3 | 4 | Pull-ups |

Cool-down

### Swimming (daily if possible)

Running warm-up

Swim continuously using the sidestroke for 10 minutes without fins.

Swim continuously using the sidestroke for 10 minutes with fins.

Running cool-down

### Running

Running warm-up

Run 3 miles at a $7^{3}/_{4}$-minute-per-mile pace; total, 9 miles per week.

Running cool-down

## WEEK 5

Warm-up

| PT | Sets | Reps | Exercise |
|---|---|---|---|
| | 6 | 25 | Push-ups |
| | 6 | 25 | Sit-ups |
| | 2 | 8 | Pull-ups |

Cool-down

### Swimming (daily if possible)

Running warm-up

Swim continuously using the sidestroke for 12 minutes without fins.

Swim continuously using the sidestroke for 12 minutes with fins.

Running cool-down

### Running

Running warm-up

Run 4 times at a $7^{3}/_{4}$-minute-per-mile pace:

    Monday—2 miles

    Tuesday— 3 miles

    Thursday— 3 miles

    Friday— 2 miles

    Total 10 miles per week

Running cool-down

## WEEK 6

Warm-up

| PT | Sets | Reps | Exercise |
|---|---|---|---|
| | 6 | 25 | Push-ups |
| | 6 | 25 | Sit-ups |
| | 2 | 8 | Pull-ups |

Cool-down

### Swimming (daily if possible)

Running warm-up

Swim continuously using the sidestroke for 12 minutes without fins.

Swim continuously using the sidestroke for 12 minutes with fins.

Running cool-down

### Running

Running warm-up

Run 4 times at a $7^{1}/_{2}$-minute-per-mile pace:

    Monday—2 miles

    Tuesday—3 miles

    Thursday— 3 miles

    Friday— 2 miles

    Total 10 miles per week

Running cool-down

## WEEK 7

Warm-up

| PT | Sets | Reps | Exercise |
|---|---|---|---|
| | 6 | 30 | Push-ups |
| | 6 | 30 | Sit-ups |
| | 2 | 10 | Pull-ups |

Cool-down

### Swimming (daily if possible)

Running warm-up

Swim continuously using the sidestroke for 10 minutes without fins.

Swim continuously using the sidestroke for 20 minutes with fins.

Running cool-down

### Running

Running warm-up

Run 4 times at a 7½-minute-per-mile pace:

    Monday—3 miles

    Tuesday—2 miles

    Friday—3 miles

    Saturday—2 miles

    Total 10 miles per week

Running cool-down

## WEEK 8

Warm-up

| PT | Sets | Reps | Exercise |
|---|---|---|---|
| | 6 | 30 | Push-ups |
| | 6 | 30 | Sit-ups |
| | 2 | 10 | Pull-ups |

Cool-down

### Swimming (daily if possible)

Running warm-up

Swim continuously using the sidestroke for 10 minutes without fins.

Swim continuously using the sidestroke for 20 minutes with fins.

Running cool-down

### Running

Running warm-up

Run 4 times at a 7½-minute-per-mile pace:

    Monday—3 miles

    Tuesday—2 miles

    Friday—3 miles

    Saturday—2 miles

    Total 10 miles per week

Running cool-down

## WEEK 9

Warm-up

| PT | Sets | Reps | Exercise |
|---|---|---|---|
| | 6 | 30 | Push-ups |
| | 6 | 30 | Sit-ups |
| | 2 | 10 | Pull-ups |

Cool-down

### Swimming (daily if possible)

Running warm-up

Swim continuously using the sidestroke for 35 minutes with fins.

Running cool-down

### Running

Running warm-up

Run 4 times at a 7½-minute-per-mile pace:

    Monday—3 miles

    Tuesday—2 miles

    Friday—3 miles

    Saturday—2 miles

    Total 10 miles per week

Running cool-down

*Note.* To skip Schedule I, successfully complete the Week 9 workout. If that week's exercise can be completed, move on to Schedule II.

## PHYSICAL TRAINING SCHEDULE II

### WEEK 1

Workout days: Monday, Wednesday, Friday
Warm-up

| PT | Sets | Reps | Exercise |
|----|------|------|----------|
|    | 6    | 30   | Push-ups |
|    | 6    | 35   | Sit-ups  |
|    | 3    | 10   | Pull-ups |
|    | 3    | 20   | Dips     |

Cool-down

*Note.* These calisthenic workouts are intended to build up long-distance muscular endurance. High-repetition workouts cause the muscles to take a longer and longer time to grow tired. Alternating exercise sets, such as doing one set of push-ups, then one set of sit-ups, and so on, will rest a given muscle group for a short time and break up the monotony of a workout.

### Swimming (daily if possible)

Running warm-up
Swim continuously using the sidestroke for 35 minutes with fins.
Running cool-down

### Running

Running warm-up
Run 4 times at a 7½-minute-per-mile pace:
>    Monday—3 miles
>    Tuesday—2 miles
>    Friday—3 miles
>    Saturday—2 miles
>    Total 10 miles per week

Running cool-down

### WEEK 2

Warm-up

| PT | Sets | Reps | Exercise |
|----|------|------|----------|
|    | 6    | 30   | Push-ups |
|    | 6    | 35   | Sit-ups  |
|    | 3    | 10   | Pull-ups |
|    | 3    | 20   | Dips     |

Cool-down

### Swimming (daily if possible)

Running warm-up
Swim continuously using the sidestroke for 35 minutes with fins.
Running cool-down

### Running

Running warm-up
Run 4 times at a 7¼-minute-per-mile pace:
>    Monday—3 miles
>    Tuesday—2 miles
>    Friday—3 miles
>    Saturday—2 miles
>    Total 10 miles per week

Running cool-down

### WEEK 3

Warm-up

| PT | Sets | Reps | Exercise |
|----|------|------|----------|
|    | 10   | 20   | Push-ups |
|    | 10   | 25   | Sit-ups  |
|    | 4    | 10   | Pull-ups |
|    | 10   | 15   | Dips     |

Cool-down

### Swimming (daily if possible)

Running warm-up
Swim continuously using the sidestroke for 45 minutes with fins.
Running cool-down

### Running

Running warm-up

Run 3 times at a 7¼-minute-per-mile pace:

    Monday—4 miles

    Thursday—4 miles

    Saturday—4 miles

    Total 12 miles per week

Running cool-down

## WEEK 4

Warm-up

| PT | Sets | Reps | Exercise |
|----|------|------|----------|
| | 10 | 20 | Push-ups |
| | 10 | 25 | Sit-ups |
| | 4 | 10 | Pull-ups |
| | 10 | 15 | Dips |

Cool-down

### Swimming (daily if possible)

Running warm-up

Swim continuously using the sidestroke for 45 minutes with fins.

Running cool-down

### Running

Running warm-up

Run 3 times at a 7-minute-per-mile pace:

    Monday—4 miles

    Thursday—4 miles

    Saturday—4 miles

    Total 12 miles per week

Running cool-down

## WEEK 5

Warm-up

| PT | Sets | Reps | Exercise |
|----|------|------|----------|
| | 15 | 20 | Push-ups |
| | 15 | 25 | Sit-ups |
| | 4 | 12 | Pull-ups |
| | 15 | 15 | Dips |

Cool-down

### Swimming (daily if possible)

Running warm-up

Swim continuously using the sidestroke for 60 minutes with fins.

Running cool-down

### Running

Running warm-up

Run 3 times at a 7-minute-per-mile pace:

    Monday—5 miles

    Thursday—2 miles

    Saturday—6 miles

    Total 13 miles per week

Running cool-down

## WEEK 6

Warm-up

| PT | Sets | Reps | Exercise |
|----|------|------|----------|
| | 20 | 20 | Push-ups |
| | 20 | 25 | Sit-ups |
| | 5 | 12 | Pull-ups |
| | 20 | 15 | Dips |

Cool-down

### Swimming (daily if possible)

Running warm-up

Swim continuously using the sidestroke for 75 minutes with fins.

Running cool-down

### Running

Running warm-up

Run 3 times at a 7-minute-per-mile pace:

    Monday—5 miles

    Thursday—3 miles

    Saturday—5 miles

    Total 13 miles per week

Running cool-down

## WEEKS 7, 8, AND 9

Warm-up

| PT | Sets | Reps | Exercise |
|---|---|---|---|
| | 20 | 20 | Push-ups |
| | 20 | 25 | Sit-ups |
| | 5 | 12 | Pull-ups |
| | 20 | 15 | Dips |

Cool-down

### Swimming (daily if possible)

Running warm-up

Swim continuously using the sidestroke for 75 minutes with fins.

Running cool-down

### Running

Running warm-up

Run 3 times at a 7-minute-per-mile pace:

Monday—2 miles

Thursday—5 miles

Saturday—6 miles

Total 13 miles per week

Running cool-down

*Note.* To skip Schedule II, successfully complete the BUD/S Screening Test as follows;

## BUD/S SCREENING TEST

1. Swim continuously 500 yards utilizing the side-stroke or the breaststroke. Pool sides may be pushed off of during turns.

Time limit—12 minutes 30 seconds

Ten-minute rest period in the standing position.

2. Perform a maximum number (minimum 42) of push-ups (see page 49) within the prescribed time.

Time limit—2 minutes

Two-minute rest period in the standing position.

3. Perform the maximum number (minimum 50) of standard sit-ups (see page 69) within the prescribed time limit.

Time limit—2 minutes

4. Perform eight continuous standard pull-ups in perfect form.

No time limit

Ten-minute rest period in the standing position.

5. Run 1½ miles while wearing full-length trousers and combat boots.

Time limit—11 minutes 30 seconds

*Note.* The above minimum exercise counts should be exceeded while taking the test.

## PHYSICAL TRAINING SCHEDULE III

## PHASE I—12 WEEKS

Day One—Total-body weight training

Day Two—1-mile swim

Day Three—Short PT/2-mile run or equivalent interval running

Day Four—Total-body weight training

Day Five—4-mile run

Day Six—Long PT/½-mile swim or interval swimming

Day Seven—Off

*Note.* Try to alternate your interval running and swimming every other week in a staggered order so that interval running and interval swimming do not take place during the same week.

### Phase I Short PT

Warm-up

| PT | Sets | Reps | Exercise |
|---|---|---|---|
| | 2 | 25 | Bent leg crunches |
| | 2 | 25 | Stomach flutter kicks |
| | 2 | 25 | Raised bent leg crunches |
| | 2 | 20 | Half sit-ups |
| | 2 | 10 | Wave-offs |

| PT | Sets | Reps | Exercise |
|----|------|------|----------|
|    | 2    | 15   | Trunk rotations |
|    | 3    | 20   | Push-ups |
|    | 2    | 15   | Lunges |
|    | 2    | 15   | Dips |
|    | 2    | 15   | Half-deep knee bends |

Cool-down

## Phase I Long PT

Warm-up

| PT | Sets | Reps | Exercise |
|----|------|------|----------|
|    | 3    | 25   | Push-ups |
|    | 4    | 25   | Bent leg crunches |
|    | 3    | 15   | Dips |
|    | 4    | 25   | Stomach flutter kicks |
|    | 2    | 12   | Hanging knee-ups, right/left side |
|    | 2    | 12   | Hanging knee-ups, straight |
|    | 2    | 12   | Eight-count body builders |
|    | 3    | 15   | Trunk rotations |
|    | 3    | 10   | Wave-offs |
|    | 2    | 12   | Lunges |
|    | 3    | 15   | Half-deep knee bends |
|    | 3    | 10   | Standard pull-ups |
|    | 3    | 10   | Wide grip pull-ups |
|    | 3    | 10   | Side-to-side pull-ups |

Cool-down

## Phase I Interval Running

Running warm-up

| Distance | Time | Rest |
|----------|------|------|
| 25 yards | 7 seconds | 1 minute |
| 50 yards | 14 seconds | 1 minute |
| 75 yards | 21 seconds | 1 minute |
| 100 yards | 28 seconds | 1 minute |

Repeat 3 times

Running cool-down

## Phase I Interval Swimming

300-meter warm-up with fins

| Sets | Distance Per Set | Time Per Set |
|------|------------------|--------------|
| 4 | 200 meters swum with fins | 4 min. 45 sec. each |
| 4 | 100 meters swum without fins | 2 min. 30 sec. each |
| 10 | 50 meters swum without fins | 1 min. 20 sec. each |

200-meter freestyle cool-down swim

## PHASE II—11 WEEKS

Day One—Total-body weight training

Day Two—1$\frac{1}{2}$- to 2-mile swim

Day Three—Long PT/4-mile run or equivalent interval running

Day Four—Total-body weight training

Day Five—8-mile run

Day Six—Short PT/$\frac{3}{4}$- to 1-mile swim or interval swimming

Day Seven—Off

*Note.* Try to alternate your interval running and swimming every other week in a staggered order so that interval running and interval swimming do not take place on the same week.

## Phase II Short PT

Warm-up

| PT | Sets | Reps | Exercise |
|----|------|------|----------|
|    | 2    | 35   | Bent leg crunches |
|    | 2    | 35   | Stomach flutter kicks |
|    | 2    | 25   | Raised bent leg crunches |
|    | 2    | 20   | Half sit-ups |
|    | 2    | 10   | Wave-offs |
|    | 2    | 18   | Trunk rotations |
|    | 3    | 25   | Push-ups |
|    | 2    | 20   | Lunges |
|    | 3    | 12   | Dips |
|    | 2    | 20   | Half-deep knee bends |

Cool-down

## Phase II Long PT

Warm-up

| PT | Sets | Reps | Exercise |
|---|---|---|---|
| | 5 | 25 | Push-ups |
| | 4 | 35 | Bent leg crunches |
| | 3 | 25 | Dips |
| | 4 | 30 | Stomach flutter kicks |
| | 3 | 12 | Hanging knee-ups, right/left side |
| | 3 | 12 | Hanging knee-ups, straight |
| | 3 | 12 | Eight-count body builders |
| | 3 | 18 | Trunk rotations |
| | 3 | 12 | Wave-offs |
| | 2 | 15 | Lunges |
| | 3 | 25 | Half-deep knee bends |
| | 3 | 12 | Standard pull-ups |
| | 3 | 12 | Wide grip pull-ups |
| | 3 | 12 | Side-to-side pull-ups |

Cool-down

## Phase II Interval Running

Running warm-up

| Distance | Time | Rest |
|---|---|---|
| 25 yards | 6 seconds | 30 seconds |
| 50 yards | 12 seconds | 30 seconds |
| 75 yards | 18 seconds | 30 seconds |
| 100 yards | 24 seconds | 30 seconds |

Repeat 4 times

Running cool-down

## Phase II Interval Swimming

300-meter warm-up with fins

| Sets | Distance Per Set | Time Per Set |
|---|---|---|
| 6 | 200 meters swum with fins | 4 min. 30 sec. each |
| 6 | 100 meters swum without fins | 2 min. 15 sec. each |
| 12 | 50 meters swum without fins | 1 min. 10 sec. each |

200-meter freestyle cool-down swim

## PHASE III—11 WEEKS

Day One—Long PT/4-mile run or equivalent interval running

Day Two—Weight training—Legs/abdominals

Day Three—Total Body Weight Training

Day Four—2-mile swim or equivalent interval swimming

Day Five—Weight Training—Legs/abdominals

Day Six—Short PT / 5- to 8-mile run

Day Seven—Off

*Note.* It is very important to discipline yourself during Schedule III, Phase III. This is the time when the mental training for BUD/S begins in earnest. If a day or two is missed from the training schedule, start again at the time where you left off; i.e., if you are on Day Three, which is a Monday, and are unable to continue the program until Thursday, you would pick up the schedule on Day Four. Try not to miss more than two days in a row. If more than two days are missed, begin the schedule again at Day One.

## WEIGHT TRAINING WORKOUTS

These are the specific exercise workouts with weights for the schedules listed above. Starting weights for weight training should be an amount that allows the completion of 3 sets of 12 repetitions of an exercise, with no more than 2 minutes' rest between sets, using the proper form and control. Increase the number of repetitions per set until 15 to 20 reps per set can be completed. When 15 to 20 reps can be completed, increase the weight for the exercise until again 3 sets of 12 reps can be just completed.

Increasing the number of repetitions for a given exercise raises the muscular endurance for the targeted muscle groups. Using a lower number

THE UNITED STATES NAVY SEALS WORKOUT GUIDE

of repetitions but a greater weight will increase the strength of the targeted muscle group. Both strength and endurance are required for BUD/S and operations within the Teams. Combining a higher number of repetitions, the exact number to be determined by the individual according to his needs, with the increase in weight balances the strength/endurance ratio for this application of weight training.

## TOTAL-BODY WEIGHT WORKOUT

Warm-up

Bench press

Overhead (military) press

Upright row

Arm (barbell) curl

Overhead (bench) triceps extension

Reverse curls

Leg press

Leg curls (knee flexions)

Leg (knee) extensions

Calf (heel) raises

Cool-down

## UPPER-BODY WEIGHT WORKOUT

Warm-up

Bench press

Overhead (military) press

Upright row

Arm (barbell) curl

Overhead (bench) triceps extension

Reverse curls

Cool-down

## LOWER-BODY WEIGHT WORKOUT

Warm-up

Leg press

Leg curls (knee flexions)

Leg (knee) extensions

Calf (heel) raises

Cool-down

## Phase III Short PT

Warm-up

| PT | Sets | Reps | Exercise |
|---|---|---|---|
| | 3 | 35 | Bent leg crunches |
| | 3 | 35 | Stomach flutter kicks |
| | 3 | 35 | Raised bent leg crunches |
| | 2 | 25 | Half sit-ups |
| | 3 | 12 | Wave-offs |
| | 3 | 15 | Trunk rotations |
| | 3 | 30 | Push-ups |
| | 2 | 25 | Lunges |
| | 3 | 15 | Dips |
| | 2 | 25 | Half-deep knee bends |

Cool-down

## Phase III Long PT

Warm-up

| PT | Sets | Reps | Exercise |
|---|---|---|---|
| | 5 | 35 | Push-ups |
| | 4 | 40 | Bent leg crunches |
| | 3 | 30 | Dips |
| | 4 | 30 | Stomach flutter kicks |
| | 3 | 15 | Hanging knee-ups, right/ left side |
| | 3 | 15 | Hanging knee-ups, straight |
| | 3 | 15 | Eight-count body builders |
| | 3 | 20 | Trunk rotations |
| | 3 | 15 | Wave-offs |
| | 3 | 20 | Lunges |
| | 3 | 30 | Half-deep knee bends |
| | 4 | 15 | Standard pull-ups |
| | 4 | 15 | Wide grip pull-ups |
| | 4 | 15 | Side-to-side pull-ups |

Cool-down

## Phase III Interval Running

Running warm-up

| Distance | Time | Rest |
|----------|------|------|
| 25 yards | 5 seconds | 30 seconds |
| 50 yards | 10 seconds | 30 seconds |
| 75 yards | 15 seconds | 30 seconds |
| 100 yards | 20 seconds | 30 seconds |

Repeat 6 times.

Running cool-down

## Phase III Interval Swimming III

300-meter warm-up with fins

| Sets | Distance Per Set | Time Per Set |
|------|------------------|--------------|
| 8 | 200 meters swum with fins | 4 min. 15 sec. each |
| 8 | 100 meters swum without fins | 2 minutes each |
| 14 | 50 meters swum without fins | 55 seconds each |

200-meter freestyle cool-down swim

# ARMY AIRBORNE PT

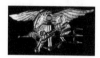

Whether it's a ten-mile swim or a ten-mile run, or even just a day of demolitions on Vieques Island, the only easy day in training is yesterday, and that's because it's over.
—SEAL, Class 28

OUTSIDE OF THE NAVY, there is one military school that all BUD/S graduates attend. That course of training is the Basic Army Airborne School at Fort Benning, Georgia. Airborne School, also called jump school, is where basic, static-line parachuting is taught, and it has long had a tradition as a difficult school in the Army. The first hour of each training day is devoted to physical training, and the balance of the day consists of at least seven more hours of rigorous training.

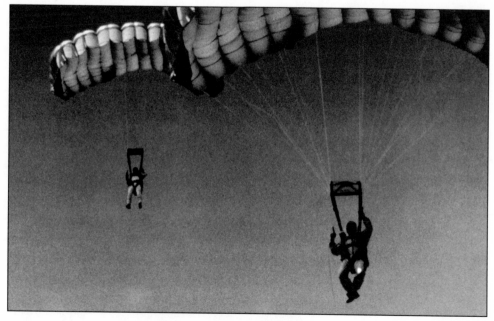

For graduates of BUD/S attending the Army school, the basic PT run at Fort Benning is considered far too light. No SEAL has ever not passed Airborne School because he couldn't do the PT. The basic idea behind the PT run at Airborne School is to build up the muscles in the legs to help cushion the shock of landing with a standard Army parachute. In addition, upper-body strength is built up along with other major muscle groups in order to help "pad out" the skeletal structure. It is far easier to operate and continue a mission with a bad bruise than with a broken bone.

Basic male daily PT at Airborne School consists of 6 chin-ups and 8 repetitions each of the following:

Side straddle hop
High jumper
Airborne sit-ups
Push-ups
Body twists
Trunk twisters
Three-quarter knee benders

Running is a constant event for the student body at Airborne School. Students are run to each classroom, event, or meal. The normal week's PT running schedule at Airborne School is:

Tuesday—2 miles in 18 minutes
Wednesday—2 miles in 18 minutes
Thursday—2½ miles in 22½ minutes
Friday—3 miles in 27 minutes

This rate of running will seem simple to BUD/S graduates. Stories have been around for years of BUD/S or earlier UDTR graduates literally running in circles around a platoon of Army Airborne students while the group was on a run. Today, a lot of the interservice rivalry once seen at service schools has been cut back considerably. PT training is also undergoing a revamping at the Army schools just as it is in the Navy as more modern and efficient techniques are brought into play.

# NUTRITION

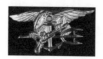

Training was what helped us complete the missions
that were given to us, and each SEALs training began
with UDTR and Hell Week. That miserable week would burn
something into the mind of each man who completed it,
something that could never be erased by time or experience.
That something was the knowledge that you could
do anything as an individual or a Team.
—SEAL, Class 28

NUTRITION IS AS important to someone undergoing physical training as the actual exercise program they are following. The body is a complex biological machine and SEAL training develops that machine into a high-performance engine. But the best engine in the world cannot run well without the proper fuel. Good nutrition will supply that fuel to the body's engine.

At BUD/S training, in the Teams, and in the Navy as a whole, good food is made available in quantity. But which items of that quantity are consumed is left up to the individual. In training as well as the Teams, excess weight due to overeating is not a great problem. The level of physical activity required of the individual just to remain qualified and in the SEALs is enough to make an overweight operator an unknown in the community.

While at BUD/S, students consume prodigious quantities of food, especially while in First Phase. During Hell Week four meals a day are offered and a student who eats 4,000 to 6,000 calories a day, and still loses weight, is hardly worth noticing. Food is simply fuel and BUD/S students are running their "engines" full out.

A problem comes with the fact that a lot of food can be consumed with little of it being nutritious. Snack and junk foods are common in our society and fast foods provide quick energy, but are not the best thing you can eat. Because these foods are common, quick, and easy, so is developing obesity, high cholesterol, and heart disease. Good nutrition focuses on what you eat, and the proportion of nutrients in the foods consumed, and not on just how much food you take in.

This section is not to be considered a weight-loss plan. It is instead a guide to a properly balanced diet. One of the normal effects of an increase in physical activity is an adjustment in an individual's weight. Thin people will tend to put on muscle tissue and gain weight, while heavier individuals may lose fat but increase their denser muscle mass. These people may remain at or near the weight they were carrying at the start of the exercise program. Truly obese people will find starting an exercise program difficult but will soon benefit from an increase in metabolism and loss of weight from their heavy concentration of body fat.

The three primary nutrients that supply energy are carbohydrates, proteins, and fats. All of these substances are burned chemically by the body to produce energy for physical activity and the body's basic maintenance. The major source of energy for short-term, high-intensity activities, such as weight training or calisthenics, are carbohydrates, preferably complex carbohydrates. Complex carbohydrates are found in foods that contain whole or enriched grain products or starches. Those foods include bread, crackers, beans, peas, rice, pasta, and starchy vegetables such as potatoes.

For the individual undergoing training, 50 to 70 percent of a day's calories should be in the form of carbohydrates. This level of carbohydrate intake can be reached by consuming the recommended 6 to 11 daily servings from the bread, cereal, rice, and pasta group; the 2 to 4 daily servings from the fruit group; and the 3 to 5 daily servings from the vegetable group.

Protein is the primary nutrient material used to build up muscle tissue. Skeletal muscle, the type

that controls movement, is made up of 22-percent protein, 70-percent water, and 7-percent fat, with the remainder being trace materials. Studies have suggested that the average body will retain up to 28 grams of protein per day from the diet and anything beyond that will go to waste.

A normal adult male requires about 0.8 gram of protein per kilogram of body weight per day. A highly active individual, such as one undergoing a physical fitness program, may have their protein needs increase slightly to 1–1.5 grams per kilogram (2.20 pounds) of body weight per day. This means that such an active individual who weighed 75 kilograms (165 pounds) would need between 75 and 113 grams of protein daily (11 to 16 ounces maximum). A recommended intake of protein would be between 10 and 15 percent of a day's total calories.

A 3-ounce portion of cooked meat, fish, or chicken supplies about 21 grams of protein. The average U.S. diet contains considerably more than 100 grams of protein per day, so the addition of such things as protein supplements in the form of powders or liquids is unnecessary at best. The necessary amount of protein required by even an active individual can be easily reached by consuming the recommended 2 to 3 daily servings from the dairy group and the 2 to 3 servings from the meat, poultry, fish, beans, eggs, and nuts group.

The remaining major nutritional group is the fats. Only about 20 to 30 percent of a day's total calories should consist of fats. In spite of the bad press given to dietary fat, the body would have a great deal of difficulty operating anywhere near peak efficiency without a sufficient amount of dietary fat. The trouble centers around the fact that the average American consumes a diet consisting of 38-percent fat. Both saturated and polyunsaturated fats should be reduced to no more than 10 percent each of a daily caloric intake. Due to the large amounts of fats found in most prepared foods, as well as those resulting from traditional cooking methods, foods from the fats, oils, and sweets group should be eaten sparingly at best.

Probably the most consistently missed nutrient is not one from any of the three major groups, but is the solvent used for all of them. The body is made up of more than 60-percent water and requires a high intake of water each day, especially when in an exercise program. Cool (40-degree) water is one of the most important items that can be consumed in a day, and yet it has no calories whatsoever.

Up to 4 quarts of water should be consumed daily. And the water should be drunk before thirst is felt. Juice, milk, soup, and other beverages all contain beneficial amounts of water but liquids containing alcohol or caffeine should be avoided as they increase the body's need for water.

A large quantity, up to 20 ounces, of water should be consumed one to two hours before exercise to promote increased hydration. This time allows the body to utilize or excrete the water as needed. During an exercise program itself, 3 to 6 ounces of water should be consumed every fifteen to thirty minutes to maintain proper hydration levels. For ease of consumption, keep a water bottle with you when working out. Fluid lost to sweat should be estimated and replaced. Losses due to sweat can be measured by the pre- and post-exercise body weights; drink 2 cups (16 ounces) of water post-exercise for each pound lost.

An individual can receive benefit from the available sports drinks when they are consumed during a long (1½ or more hours) period of intense exercise. Drinks used should contain between 5 and 10 percent carbohydrates for maximum benefit. This level of carbohydrates can provide an increase in the available energy to muscles undergoing work. Most beverages that exceed 10-percent carbohydrate content, including a majority of soft drinks and fruit juices, can have detrimental effects during an exercise program. Abdominal cramps, nausea, and diarrhea have all been reported by individuals who have consumed high-carbohydrate drinks during training.

The chart on page 164 details the various food groups, what their preferred components are, and what a serving consists of.

The materials and amounts in the chart will make up a balanced diet. Certain foods contain higher amounts of specific nutrients than others (bananas, potassium; citrus, vitamin C; milk, calcium, etc.). In a normal diet, the blend of different fruits, vegetables, and other foods will supply the vitamins and trace elements the body requires.

Vitamin or mineral supplements are usually unnecessary when a proper variety of foods are eaten. Excess vitamins and other supplements are excreted by the body and noticeable in a yellow and "chemical-smelling" urine. There are no known advantages in consuming very large amounts of any known nutrient and are known risks in taking an excess of some vitamins and trace elements. Fads come and go while good nutrition is permanent.

| FOOD GROUPS | PREFERENCE | SERVING |
|---|---|---|
| Meat, Poultry, Fish, Beans, Eggs, and Nuts | Lean cuts of meat with the fat trimmed<br>Poultry with the skin removed<br>Dry roasted nuts<br>Eggs with no yolks | 2–3 oz. meat (cooked)<br>1 egg<br>½ cup beans (cooked) |
| Dairy Products | Skim, 1%, or nonfat milk<br>Cheeses with less than 2–6 grams of fat per ounce<br>Low-fat yogurt and soft cheeses like cottage cheese | 1 cup (8 oz.) milk or yogurt<br>1½–2-oz. cheese (2 or 3 sandwich-sized slices) |
| Fruits | Raw fruit items (apple, pear, banana, orange, etc.)<br>Juice, canned or cooked fruit (lite) in juice not syrup | 1 medium fruit<br>½ grapefruit<br>¼ small melon<br>½ cup canned/cooked |
| Vegetables | Dark green, leafy, or yellow whole; raw or cooked; juice | ½ cup raw<br>1 cup leafy<br>½ cup cooked<br>1 med. potato<br>¾ cup juice |
| Breads, Cereals, Rice, Pasta, and Peas | Whole-wheat breads<br>Muffins<br>Ready-to-eat cereals (low sugar) | 1 slice<br>½ bun /muffin<br>1 oz. dry cereal |
| Fats and Oils | Unsaturated and vegetable oils<br>Margarine<br>Low-fat salad dressings | 6 to 8 teaspoonfuls daily |

# TEAMWORK

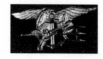

*"Do we have any individuals in here?"*
*"Negative, Master Chief. HOOYAH!"*
*—BUD/S Class 214*

*But it was the strain and just physical work of a patrol*
*like this that proved out just why most of our training involved*
*physical workouts. If we hadn't been in shape, we could have*
*never completed an op like this one, or probably*
*even survived given what happened.*
*—SEAL, Class 28*

THE TEAMS—that is the term used by the men of the U.S. Navy Special Warfare community, known to the public as the Navy SEALs. Individuals are in the Teams, or they have served in the Teams, a unique brotherhood of accomplished individuals who have one overriding thing in common—they are all Teammates.

Though incredible individual effort can be required from any one man, it is as a Team that the SEALs accomplish their objectives. A telling phrase has been heard throughout the arduous SEAL training course for decades: There is no "I" in SEAL Team.

It is as an individual that a man faces BUD/S, and it is by reaching down deep inside himself that he finds what is necessary to keep going with his class. But, it is as a member of a team that a man completes BUD/S. No matter what your preparation, there are evolutions (exercises) that you cannot complete as an individual. Log PT, IBS drill, and many other evolutions cannot be completed except by a coordinated effort from everyone involved. It is through these evolutions that the individual learns to become part of a Team and earns the right to be a member of the Special Warfare community.

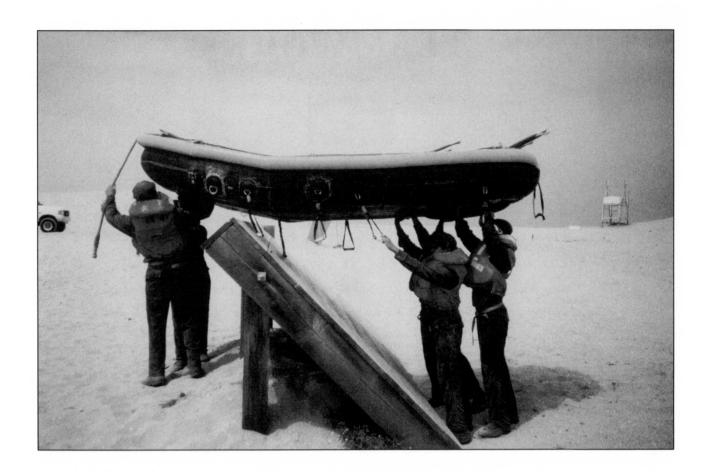

During BUD/S training, every future SEAL's strengths will be brought out and built up. At the same time, his weaknesses will be exposed and overcome. Sometimes those weaknesses are not beaten by the individual alone, but by the support and work of his classmates. During the most exhausting part of training, it is common to see one classmate reach out to help another who is falling. From the depths of his own exhaustion, one man will pull up another whose legs have temporarily failed him. That same falling man may later help his teammate lift an obstacle when his arms fail him. Each depends on the other to make the whole.

Nowhere in the Navy will the distinction between officers and enlisted men become more blurred than in BUD/S. Officers are not only expected to crawl through the mud and water alongside their men; they are expected to lead them through and out of it. If anything, training for an officer-student is that much harder; to lead by example is the only accepted way in the Teams.

This level of equality and teamwork is not created easily, nor does it come naturally. It takes a high development of self-image or ego to get an individual through BUD/S training. That same ego is suppressed for the benefit of the Teams and Teammates. The concept of Teamwork is drilled into each graduate of BUD/S and is taken with them to the Teams. The success of the SEALs is

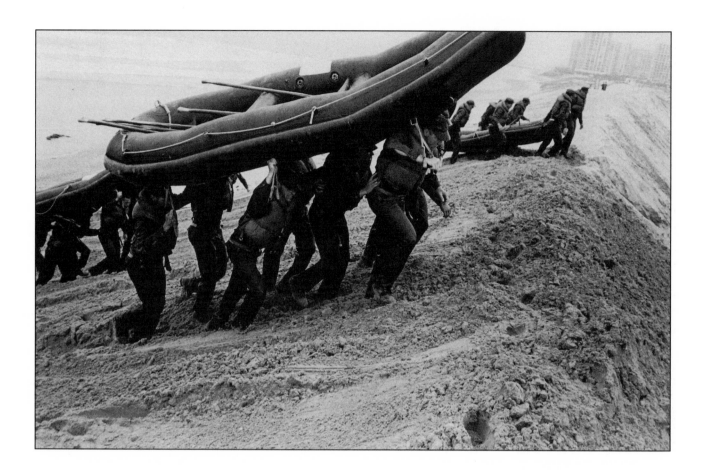

built on the efforts of a Team, and that is in turn made up of Teammates. Part of that philosophy is demonstrated by the fact that no SEAL, living or dead, has ever been left behind by his Teammates.

Only through the combined abilities and skills of a group of SEALs can many missions be accomplished. An individual would not only disrupt a Team; he could easily become a very real danger to the group. The "me-first" attitude is not allowed to exist in the Teams, and it is first weeded out during training.

# MOTIVATION

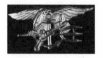

Once you completed training and entered a Team,
you were a Teammate for life. You knew what
you were and were proud of it.
**—SEAL, Class 58**

THE KEY TO completing BUD/S training is the proper preparation of the individual before arrival. The physical portion of the course can be addressed by the exercise regimens offered in this book, but the most important attribute for successful training can only come from within the individual himself. Even though it is the most physically demanding course available in the U.S. military, many SEALs who have completed BUD/S will say the same thing: "BUD/S is ten percent physical and ninety percent mental."

That statement does not say that BUD/S is not telling on the body. It requires all that a body can do and more. But the demands on the mind and the motivation of the individual are vastly greater than even the most difficult of the exercises and evolutions. Without the heart, drive, and desire to complete the course, even the most fit cannot reach graduation. The most valuable attribute a student can show up with at Coronado is what is called the "fire in the gut."

# VOLUNTEERING FOR BUD/S

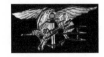

**What you can say for Hell Week is that,
in a way you get stronger as those miserable days crawl by.
More and more, as you just keep going, the resolve to
complete the course just continues to grow in you.**
**—SEAL, Class 58**

INDIVIDUALS WHO are presently enlisted in the Navy and wish to volunteer for BUD/S need to follow the procedures listed for in-service BUD/S candidates. The requirements and procedures for the BUD/S training application are:

1. Passing the BUD/S Screening Test as shown at the end of Physical Training Schedule II (see page 153)
2. Pass a diving physical examination. This exam is more stringent than regular physical evaluations.
3. Meet vision standards. Your vision must be correctable to 20/20 and no worse than 20/40 in one eye and 20/70 in the other eye with no color blindness.
4. Have a good overall performance record. Evaluations of 3.6 or higher are needed.
5. Have your 1306/7 endorsed by your commanding officer.
6. Have a minimum Armed Services Vocational Aptitude, Basic (ASVAB) score: VE + AR = 104, MC = 50.
7. Have a SEAL source rating (see page 175) or be willing to convert to a qualified source rating within one year of graduation from BUD/S.
8. Have sufficient minimum obligated time in service remaining. You must have 36 months of obligated service remaining on your class convening date. You may extend/reenlist to make up the proper time.
9. You must be 28 years old or less.
10. Only men are eligible.

Procedures:

1. Put in a "Special Request Chit" through your chain of command requesting BUD/S training.
2. Submit a "Personnel Action Request" (Form 1306/7) to SPECWAR/ Diver assignment. Submit the following with your request:
   a. A certified copy of your ASVAB test scores.
   b. Your BUD/S Screening Test results
   c. Pressure and oxygen tolerance test results (if completed}
   d. Your completed diving physical (Form SF88-SF93)
   e. Certified copy of your latest performance evaluation report

For the proper location to mail your completed package, or to receive further information of the BUD/S program call: 1-888-USN-SEAL.

At that number you will access a recorded message that will guide you to further information.

For civilians wishing to join the Navy and volunteer for the SEALs, see your local Navy recruiter or call 1-888-USN-SEAL.

# AFTERWORD

It is often said that BUD/S is the most physically demanding course in our military and perhaps in the world. Having been a BUD/S instructor for three years and the Commanding Officer for two, I can assure you that this is the case. The Naval Special Warfare Center is on a constant quest to increase our number of BUD/S graduates without lowering our standards. The best way to do that is to start with better candidates. This book goes a long way in helping that effort by explaining the BUD/S program to potential volunteers and helping them prepare for the physical rigors of BUD/S.

The majority of students who leave BUD/S do so voluntarily. They get mentally defeated, start telling themselves that they just aren't up to the task, then voluntarily disenroll—a decision that many of them regret for a long time. It's easy to get mentally defeated when you finish a day of training physically exhausted. Those students who graduate are the ones who have prepared themselves physically, well beyond the limits established in the BUD/S screening test. They end each day not so physically exhausted and with a positive attitude to continue on.

Potential candidates who will follow the guidelines of this book and push themselves prior to BUD/S will, no doubt, stand a better chance of graduating. Set your goal to graduate, prepare yourself physically, and let nothing stand in your way. With the proper physical preparation and "never say quit" attitude you stand the chance to be among the few who call themselves SEALs.

—JOE YARBOROUGH, Captain, U.S.N.

# SEAL SOURCE RATINGS

To volunteer and be acceptable to BUD/S, an enlisted Navy man has to be either classified in, or a designated striker for, the following ratings:

BM    Boatswain's Mate
EM    Electrician's Mate
EN    Engineman
ET    Electronics Technician
GMG   Gunner's Mate—Guns
GMM   Gunner's Mate—Missiles
HM    Hospital Corpsman
HT    Hull Maintenance Technician
IC    Interior Communications Electrician
IS    Intelligence Specialist
MM    Machinist's Mate
MN    Mineman
MR    Machinery Repairman
OS    Operations Specialist

OT    Ocean Systems Technician
PH    Photographer's Mate
PN    Personnelman
PR    Survival Aircrew Equipmentman
QM    Quartermaster
RM    Radioman
SK    Storekeeper
SM    Signalman
STG   Sonar Technician
TM    Torpedoman Mate
WT    Weapons Technician
YN    Yeoman

Volunteers who are applying for the BUD/S program from within the Navy must sign a "page 13" entry agreeing to convert to an approved SEAL source rating within one year after training.

# GLOSSARY

**Aerobic**  An exercise that raises and maintains the heart rate at a high level and requires breathing in large volumes of air.

**Barbell**  A long bar with room for both hands in the center and removable weights on both ends.

**BUD/S**  Basic Underwater Demolition/SEAL training. Considered the toughest course of instruction in the U.S. military, these twenty-six weeks of training must be completed by everyone who wishes to become a SEAL. There are no shortcuts; you have either completed the full course or you haven't.

**Circuit**  A series of exercises in a workout. The series may be intended to target a specific area of the body or obtain a general workout over the entire body.

**Closed-Circuit Training**  The specialized UBA (underwater breathing apparatus) training received by BUD/S students The closed-circuit system, also called a rebreather, is the primary UBA used in all of the SEAL Teams.

**Drownproofing**  A course of training that must be passed by all BUD/S students. Drownproofing involves dangerous exercises performed in the water under the constant supervision of the BUD/S instructors. The student learns how to maintain his buoyancy, control panic, and survive in the water under adverse circumstances.

**Dumbbell**  A short bar with weights on both ends intended to be held with one hand. The dumbbell may be adjustable with removable weights or be in one piece and a fixed weight.

**Free Weights**  Weights in the form of barbells, dumbbells, and other movable objects used to give resistance to muscle movement while exercising. Free weights are normally held by the hands or body with no other external support. This allows a more dynamic motion to the exercise, involving not only movement of the weight but also maintaining balance and coordinating the use of the arms, legs, and whatever portions of the body are needed for the support of the exercise.

**Hydrographic Surveys** The original mission of the UDTs, or frogmen, of World War II. A hydrographic reconnaissance measures the depth of the water, contours of the sea bottom, and locates obstacles from the twenty-one-foot depth line to the high-water mark on the beach. A survey is conducted by a group of swimmers, spaced out at twenty-five-foot intervals, who swim in to the beach, measuring the water and making notes on plastic slates.

**Isotonic Training** This form of exercise requires the movement of the body against a resistance. An isotonic contraction is one where the muscle contracts and shortens while movement is taking place. Whenever an individual does a calisthenic exercise or moves a weight, an isotonic contraction takes place.

**PT** The military abbreviation for physical training.

**Rebreather** An underwater breathing system where the breathing gases are moved in and out of a flexible bag as the operator breathes. The exhaled gases are scrubbed chemically of carbon dioxide, and pure oxygen is injected into the system to make up for what was consumed by the swimmer. To prevent difficulties, the breathing medium used in the standard rebreather is pure oxygen. Pure oxygen becomes toxic when used at too high a pressure, so the depth at which a rebreather is used must be constantly monitored. The lack of exhaust bubbles and the difficulty of tracking underwater a swimmer who is using a rebreather are what make the system valuable to Naval Special Warfare.

**Red Cell** A special classified unit of men put together in the Navy to test security on naval installations.

**Repetition (Rep)** A single complete movement of an exercise, not including picking up or setting down a weight or getting into position.

**Routine** The group of sets done for a particular movement.

**Scuba Diving** Swimming underwater using self-contained underwater breathing apparatus, also called UBA in the Teams. Scuba uses compressed air as the breathing medium. The air is inhaled through a regulator that adjusts the pressure to match that of the surrounding water. Once the air is exhaled, it escapes into the water as a cloud of bubbles, which can betray the location of a scuba swimmer. Normal scuba gear is also referred to as open-circuit UBAs in the SEALs.

**SDV Teams** Or SEAL Delivery Vehicle Teams. The SDVTs operate small underwater craft that can move a number of SEAL operators and their equipment for long distances underwater without being detected. An SDV operator is a fully qualified SEAL whose mission can require him to be isolated underwater in the cold and dark for hours at a time. There are two SDV Teams, Team One in Hawaii and Team Two in Little Creek, Virginia.

**SEAL Teams** The basic operational units of Naval Special Warfare. A SEAL Team is a group of operational platoons, each of which can work independently of the others according to mission requirements. There are seven SEAL Teams, numbered One through Eight (less Seven). Odd-numbered SEAL Teams are stationed on the West Coast in Coronado, California, and even-numbered SEAL Teams are on the East Coast at Little Creek, Virginia.

**Set**  The number of repetitions done in a single sequence with no rest between them as part of a workout routine.

**Special Operations (DOD)**  Operations conducted by specially trained, equipped, and organized Department of Defense forces against strategic or tactical targets in pursuit of national military, political, economic, or psychological objectives. These operations may be conducted during periods of peace or hostilities. They may support conventional operations, or they may be prosecuted independently when the use of conventional forces is either inappropriate or infeasible.

**Special Warfare**  The official Navy term for the SEALs.

**Team**  To any past or present member of Naval Special Warfare, the Team is always capitalized and is used to indicate the SEAL Team.

**Total Body Weight Training**  Weight training in which each part of the body is worked through a series of exercises as compared to just working out on the legs, arms, abdominals, et cetera.

**UDTR**  Underwater Demolition Team Replacement training, the original basic course that all members of the UDTs or SEALs had to complete to enter the Teams. The term was changed to BUD/S in the early 1970s when SEAL training was included in the course.

# INDEX

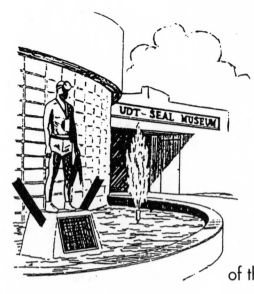

# UDT-SEAL MUSEUM

...Located on the Original Training Site
of the Navy Frogmen in Fort Pierce, Florida

The UDT-SEAL Museum tells the story of U.S. Navy special warfare from the early days of Naval Combat Demolition Units and Scouts & Raiders to Underwater Demolition Teams—better known as Frogmen—and today's SEALs. Outdoor and indoor exhibits illustrate the unique history of the men who fought in World War II, and those who followed them in Korea and Vietnam. Also part of the exhibits are recent operations in Haiti, Somalia, and Iraq.

The museum, dedicated to preserving the weapons, equipment, artifacts, vehicles, and valor of the country's most secretive fighting men, is operated by the UDT-SEAL Museum Association. For information about becoming an association member, contact the association at the address below, or call (561) 595-1570, or fax (561) 595-1576.

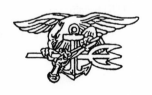

UDT-SEAL Museum
3300 North A1A
North Hutchinson Island
Fort Pierce, FL 34949-8520
(561) 462-3597

# ABOUT THE AUTHORS

**Master Chief Boatswain's Mate Dennis Chalker, U.S.N. (Ret.)**

Time spent in the Army with the 82nd Airborne, college, and a long career with Navy Special Warfare show that Dennis Chalker has "been there and done that." Assignments to SEAL Team One, and as a plank owner of SEAL Team Six and Red Cell illustrate the capabilities of Master Chief Chalker better than any list of decorations or accomplishments, of which he has many. As the Master Chief of the Command for the Naval Special Warfare Center, Training Group, Dennis Chalker well knows what it takes to be a SEAL and shares his knowledge on these pages.

**Kevin Dockery**

Fourteen years in military service well prepared Kevin Dockery for his present involvement with the Navy Special Warfare community. As the author of *SEALs in Action, Point Man, Walking Point, The Teams,* and *Special Warfare—Special Weapons,* among other works, Kevin has demonstrated his ability to properly tell the story of the Teams.

**Deverick T. Lampley**

Deverick Lampley was a consultant for *The United States Navy SEALs Workout Guide.* Numerous track honors and awards in college demonstrate his athletic abilities. His qualifying for the 1996 Olympic time trials and signing with the Dallas Cowboys (1985) and Tampa Bay Buccaneers (1986) as a free agent show that his abilities are far above the norm. As a fully qualified personal trainer and owner of the Bodies Plus Fitness Center in Huntington Beach, California, Deverick is well experienced in bringing a fit way of life and a proper training regimen to the general public.